THE
Amazing
HEALING
POWER OF
Kitchari

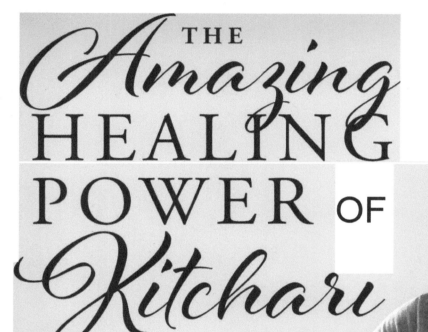

Weight Loss

Anti-inflammatory

Soup

Dr. Shasta Ericson L.Ac., D.A.O.M.

Acknowledgments

I'd like to dedicate this book to my son, Kai. I wish him a wonderful life filled with joy and peace.

I'd like to acknowledge my yoga teacher, Baba Hari Dass, for sharing kitchari with me and for being the biggest inspiration in my life. I'd also like to acknowledge Darlena La'Orange L.Ac. for teaching me most of what I know about Kitchari, Lesley Birch, my coach, Chris Welsh, and my friends Ralph Houghton, Hillari Dowdle, Farnaz Tehrani, Brittney O'Brien, Dr. Mark Bergmann, Hema Munshi, Monica Espinoza, Ann Roman, Shannon Ty Arriaga, and Judy Specht for always encouraging and supporting me. John Sanchez and Noella Vigeant for the photographs, and all of my patients and my two students, Sarah Fields L.Ac. and Jacki Brown L.Ac. who generously shared their experiences and recipes for this book.

Special thank you to Lakeisha Ethans for helping make this book come true!

Disclaimer

No part of this publication may be reproduced or transmitted in any form or by any means, electronic or mechanical, including photo-copying, recording or by any information storage and retrieval system, without written permission from the author, except for the inclusion of brief quotations in a review.

All products and/or services mentioned in this publication bearing the name, likeness, or image of any other company or product line are trademarks, registered trademarks, or service marks of the respective companies identified. No endorsement or approval by such companies is or should be inferred by their inclusion herein. The author is not affiliated with, or endorsed by, Google Inc. in any manner.

The author has put forth a best effort in ensuring the content of this publication is accurate and current as of the time of publication. The author is not responsible for any inadvertent errors, omissions, or contrary interpretations of the subject matter herein. The author makes no warranty of any kind, expressed or implied, with regard to the information supplied.

No guarantees are made. The author shall not be liable in the event of incidental or consequential damages in connection with, or arising out of, the providing of information offered herein. The author is not responsible for external changes that may affect the applicability of

Table of Contents

Introduction

MY YOGA TEACHER Baba Hari Dass (called Babaji) said that the yogis in India eat kitchari as it's a complete meal nourishing all aspects of the body. According to Babaji, the word "kitchari" is made up of two words: *khe*—sky and *chari*—walk, i.e., skywalk or walking in the sky—perhaps because kitchari digests so easily that it makes you feel as light as air. Babaji says that the yogis in India eat the kitchari daily as they believe it is a complete, healthy meal.

Many people have struggled most of their lives trying to maintain a healthy weight, and as a second-generation doctor of acupuncture, oriental medicine, and a wellness coach with over twenty-five years in clinical practice, I have counseled thousands of people about their weight. If you're having a difficult time controlling your weight, you may be somewhat happy to learn more about this ancient Ayurvedic medicinal cleansing soup.

According to the CDC's most recent survey of Americans' health, almost 32 percent of the two- to nineteen-year-olds and nearly 69 percent of all adults in America are overweight or obese (Hoffman & Salerno, 2012, p. 11). In the article published by *Acupuncture Today*, Bruce H. Robinson, MD says, "The figures that verify this crisis are astounding. In 1985, less than 10 percent of Americans were obese and about the same percentage were significantly overweight, for a total of about 20 percent. Now, in 2013, the combined total of those overweight or obese has reached 74 percent, according to the World Health Organization, with about half of these individuals overweight and the other half obese. All of these individuals are at increased risk for developing diabetes, as well as acquiring hypertension, heart disease, cancer and strokes" (Robinson, 2013, p. 18).

Complications of obesity in the US cause as many as 300,000 premature deaths each year, making it second only to cigarette smoking as a preventable cause of death. Complications of obesity are: 1) Metabolic syndrome, 2) diabetes mellitus, 3) cardiovascular disease, 4) nonalcoholic steatohepatitis (fatty liver), 5) gallbladder disease, 6) gastro esophageal reflux, 7) obstructive sleep apnea, 8) reproductive system disorders, 9) many cancers, 10) osteoarthritis and, 11) social and psychological problems (Porter & Kaplan, 2011, p. 56-57).

Almost all cases of obesity result from a combination of genetic predisposition and a chronic imbalance between energy intake, energy utilization for basic metabolic processes, and energy expenditure from physical activity.

Diagnosis usually is done through body mass index (BMI), waist circumference, and sometimes body composition analysis, which includes fat caliper testing (Porter & Kaplan, 2011, p. 58). This may sound like "a calorie in is a calorie to be burned"; however, new research is finding that a calorie is not just a calorie. As Dr. Mark Hyman states, "Food that enters your bloodstream quickly promotes weight gain; food that enters slowly promotes weight loss" (Hyman, M., 2006, p. 22). Another issue is psychological, as people who are overweight or obese may feel pressure to look normal, and this can lead to poor self-esteem and even an inability to participate in normal daily activities, resulting in mental, physical, and spiritual stress.

Stress and other lifestyle factors such as proper sleep are very important for maintaining a healthy weight. According to Chris D'Adamo, PhD, "It is important to consider stress management. There is strong evidence showing that people who are stressed may experience weight gain, as can those with sleep deprivation or poor sleep hygiene" (Ulbricht, D'Adamo, Edman, & Ernst, 2011, p. 83). Diet therapy, a part of Complementary and Alternative Medicine (CAM), aims to create balance, a point of integrity of the body, mind, and spirit, and enhance resilience. Self-care with diet therapy has an added benefit of less financial cost, which contributes to less stress. D'Adamo states, "With an increase of stress hormones, such as cortisol, epinephrine, and norepinephrine, this may lead to increased blood sugar" (Ulbricht, et al, 2011, p. 83).

If you're reading this you know how painful it is to fall prey to the fatal attraction of food. Just like you, I went through a number of diets, all of which worked as long as I stuck with them. The moment "diet fatigue" set in, I fell off the wagon and gained back whatever weight I had earlier lost and more. I'm sure you've also experienced similar things in your diet journey, but here's where we differ.

Being a professional in my career, I have access to a lot of information relating to natural weight loss and detoxification. I also have learned that proper nutrition affects longevity, health, and mental state of happiness. As you read on I hope you will be encouraged to try kitchari, as it is good for detoxification and weight loss and overall metabolism. Once you understand everything that I have to give you, I hope you will have all the motivation you need to begin losing weight and improving your own health for the rest of your life.

In discussing various subjects related to health, slimness, and longevity, I have offered advice on diet, nutrition, and the important role of food in human life. Remember that proper diet is the key factor behind amazing signs of physical improvement.

Those who practice how to eat the right foods will notice improvement in their health simply because the burden on their digestive system has lessened. Eating the right food not only contributes to weight loss but also leaves you with a great digestive system, energy, and overall good health. When I say weight loss I literally mean you looking forward to those early morning trips to the bathroom scale! Soon you will notice that the excess pounds, hip-hugging fat, jiggly arms, and puckered cellulite will burn away faster than you thought possible.

Think about it like this; if your digestive system is up to mark, you will no longer require large amounts of water to flush out dead cells, and thus you will not get bloated from fluid retention—leading you to be slimmer and trimmer. There are many people who seek to lose twenty to fifty pounds quickly in hopes of attending an upcoming wedding or going on a trip to the beach with the perfect body.

My plan is not a crash diet, and like many healthier individuals would agree, a crash diet is not the best way to shed some pounds, as 95 percent of these diets fail, mainly due to the lack of high-nutrient-value foods. My plan is healthier and is meticulously designed to supply nutrition while allowing an individual to lose weight quickly. The best part about my plan is that, for those who exercise regularly, this plan can be coupled with exercise programs for amazing results.

Let's try something here for a minute. Try to picture yourself in remarkable health and tremendous physical condition, at your ideal body weight. Not only will your body be free of fat, but your heart will also be free of burden. When you look at what you want to achieve and where you are now, the road seems somewhat blurry. Of course it is not easy to change your eating habits, simply because eating has emotional and social relations. As you will discover, our American diet style is addictive, and why not? The smell of burgers and the cheese from pizzas—who would that not lure! Every single day you have hundreds of choices to make about what you put into your body, but it is important to remember that changing the way you eat may not happen overnight.

Let me assure you that many people have tried what I have to offer, and to their surprise, after they adopted the change, they found that their life was much easier, they were more energetic, and what they ate was more delicious than ever before. As your health improves, so will your taste buds and eventually you will learn to love the healthy food you eat. Of course it takes time to create new food preferences, but I guarantee you that the wait will be worth your time. Making a change is not easy.

Millions of people already know that if they change their diet and get enough exercise, they can lose weight. But if you walk down the street, you still see overweight or obese people paving the way and marching to their destinations. Therefore, change is never easy; you need to be completely determined to make that happen, and only then will you see significant results in your weight, health, and overall physique.

Let me take this opportunity to thank you, my readers, for beginning the journey to wellness, or for including this in your already healthy lifestyle. I sincerely appreciate each and every individual who takes a step forward to build a healthy future, and I am committed to your success. I hope that this book inspires you to live a healthy lifestyle. I do realize that this goal may look hard to achieve at first, but the benefits of feeling healthy, being a healthy weight, and having a happy disposition are worth more than all the riches in the world.

I welcome you to the wisdom of the ancient medicines and encourage you to put this knowledge to work for your benefit.

About The Author

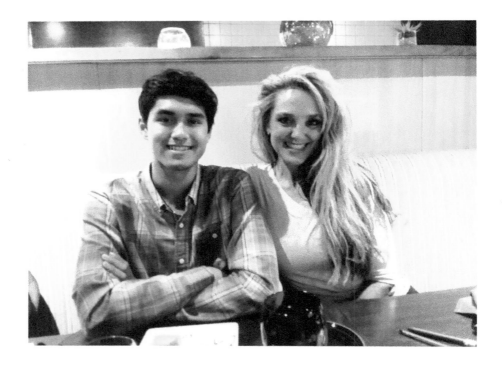

Dr. Shasta Ericson L.Ac., D.A.O.M.

Shasta Ericson is a second-generation licensed acupuncturist, natural medicine expert, and a doctor of acupuncture and oriental medicine. She is a certified yoga instructor and a wellness coach in the State of California. She has been practicing natural functional medicine and acupuncture at the Way of Wellness Natural Healthcare Inc. clinic in San Jose, California, for 25 years.

For more information on other books & courses from Dr. Shasta, specializes in general health, infertility, weight loss and pain management.

Ericson: www.kitchari.net

More here: www.WayOfWellness.com

Testimonials

"My intestinal problem has gone away. Diarrhea. They kept telling me I was lactose intolerant but I had gotten rid of all the lactose and I still had the problem. So eating this has taken care of that. I had this problem for three to four years. I would get up sometimes five or six times a night till I was completely emptied out. I stated eating the kitchari Saturday night and I haven't had a problem since. I have dropped seven pounds this week, but that is probably because that's all I've eaten…"– **Tiffany**

"I had been suffering from severe hot flashes during menopause. I was getting them every two hours, which made it almost impossible to sleep. Due to my lack of sleep I was unable to control my emotions, especially crying and depression. Shasta put me on the kitchari diet and within about six weeks I no longer had hot flashes (less than two times a week and I only feel warm), and am able to sleep six hours without waking up. My emotions are now under control and I've lost about seven pounds. I still eat the kitchari to keep my energy." – **Keye**

"I started gaining confidence and because my body was feeling better. I've lost eighteen pounds in eight weeks and now I find that I've *really started standing up for myself a lot more and not allowing my-self to be pushed around or controlled like I was previously. I now find myself feeling more in control of my food choices as well..."* – **Linda**

"I had severe sciatica due to three herniated discs in my low back which my M.D. wanted to fuse together. I was in so much pain that I could hardly walk. I was also forty-five pounds overweight. With Shasta's advice I went on the kitchari cleanse and learned about what foods were more appropriate for my constitution and symptoms, and little by little my body began to heal. Within ten months I've lost forty-five pounds, the pain is gone, I run for up to one hour on the beach, and surf like I did when I was twenty. I truly believe that when we do what's good for the body, and stop what's bad, the body will heal itself. We just have to get out of its way."
– **Robin**

Shasta's Background, Vision, & Commitment

MY NAME IS Shasta and I am a second-generation doctor of acupuncture and oriental medicine with over twenty years in clinical practice. I'm also a certified yoga instructor and a certified wellness coach. This book has been a dream of mine for the last twenty years. I wrote this because the Ayurvedic Detox Diet (with kitchari) has literally saved my life. Those who know me now may find it difficult to believe, but when I was in my twenties, I was very ill and almost died from Hashimoto's hypothyroidism, an autoimmune disease. I have person- ally experienced the profound healing available through kitchari.

I struggled with my weight the entire first half of my life. Kitchari helped me feel good and maintain my normal weight even with a sluggish metabolism. Since then I have prescribed kitchari to many patients, friends, and family members for the purpose of increasing their health and well-being—with amazing results. Out of all the natural health and self-healing strategies I have come across, kitchari makes the most difference to my health. It is the food that I still eat for at least one meal each and every day as it allows me to remain a healthy and productive person. It is my intention that you and your loved ones experience the incredible healing power of kitchari and rejuvenate your mind, body, and spirit.

My commitment to you if you follow this program is to help you lose weight, detox, and feel great in your body so that you live a life you love and fulfill your purpose in the world. I feel that since I've been given a second chance at life, it is part of my mission to offer you the tools of health that I have been blessed to discover so that you can experience the great joy of fulfilling your potential! Before I get into that though, I will share a little about my upbringing and background and how I was introduced to kitchari. I grew up on a nature commune in California in the seventies. My parents named me Shasta Free. Yes, I was a hippie kid. It was a cultural revolution. We lived close to nature, kind of how it was about a hundred years ago.

Our water came right out of the creek. We had no electricity or television; we used kerosene lamps. I was born at home and everyone I knew was born at home. Our food was naturally grown and home cooked. We raised goats and chickens. We ate goat's milk and goat's cheese and everything was cooked on woodstoves. We ate a lot of rice and beans and vegetables (which is basically what kitchari is) and the people on the commune were very healthy. We didn't go to Western doctors, unless we were very sick with ailments like pneumonia, staph infections, and broken bones. I grew up near an American Indian reservation, and Native herbs were used for many common ailments such as cold and flu.

I realize now that we had the best food and the best water in the world, and this probably helped us avoid Western medicine doc- tors for most ailments. I was fortunate enough to be introduced to Baba Hari Dass ("Babaji"), a yogi from India, when I was four. Later, Baba Hari Dass became my yoga teacher. As part of his program, his students ate kitchari for cleansing the body, mind, and spirit during weeklong yoga retreats. Now I realize how truly fortunate I was to have grown up on the nature commune and be part of the yoga com- munity, and Babaji's amazing teaching and healthy food, including the kitchari. At the age of fourteen, my food world changed.

I entered high school and was introduced to the Standard American Diet. I was amazed at all the sugary, fried foods and refined carbohydrates my classmates ate. But it wasn't until I moved to New York City at the age of twenty-one that my health problems began. I ate the Standard American Diet and within six months, I had gained thirty pounds, felt exhausted, and was always hungry. I ate mostly breads and bagels, cream cheese, spaghetti, and pizza because they were easy, quick, and cheap. In New York City you could order whatever you wanted from the local grocery store and the couriers would walk your order right up to your desk.

I'd usually order a bagel a couple times a day because that's what I could afford. I noticed that eating these processed foods made me a slave to my food, food that wasn't good for me. I had never experienced addiction to food like this before. When I was twenty-one, I moved back to California and enrolled in a three-week yoga teacher training under the guidance of Baba Hari Dass at Mount Madonna Center. Students were taught all eight limbs of ashtanga yoga, from meditation, sadhana, asanas, and panchakarma. Yoga is a part of Ayurveda, the ancient science of Indian medicine that includes dietary and lifestyle suggestions, bodywork, herbal remedies, and more.

During the yoga training, students ate whole, organic food and a bowl of kitchari at least once a day. I noticed immediately that my cravings for sugary, salty, fatty foods went away, and I lost ten pounds during the training. I was desperate to lose the remaining twenty pounds, so I asked Babaji how to do it. He said, "Just do your yoga." From his remark I realized that if I felt reconnected to the divine life force that flows through me through my practice of yoga, my mind, body, and spirit would gravitate toward health and harmony and I would naturally choose foods and lifestyle practices that would allow me to lose the extra weight and be healthy again.

I went home, cooked large pots of kitchari, and continued my Ayurvedic detox diet program for another month. I ate kitchari for two to three meals a day along with other healthy foods (fruits, nuts, and a little bit of organic animal protein) and lost the remaining twenty pounds within one month. The healthy food, yoga, and exercise routine revived my energy and my enthusiasm for life, and I discovered my life purpose: helping people have lives they love, make their dreams come true, and have a body to support them to do this... I then enrolled in Chinese medicine to begin my training for my life purpose—being a healer.

Unfortunately, hypothyroidism, which I was genetically predisposed to, crept up and by the time I was twenty-seven, I felt very unwell.

I didn't understand what was going on because I always used to feel good. I became anemic. I developed insomnia, fibromyalgia, chronic fatigue, and I had a brain fog. Back then I didn't know that I had hypothyroidism. I had suspected it because everyone in my immediate family had it, but I was repeatedly misdiagnosed by my medical doctor. As my disease progressed I began to complain about being cold most of the time. Furthermore, I couldn't lift five pounds without aggravating a torn muscle in my shoulder that refused to heal. During the prime of my life, my doctor placed me on disability and I was only allowed to work part time.

I felt so frustrated and betrayed by my body! I suffered for seven years because lab tests did not indicate clear hypothyroidism. (Since then, the test range for hypothyroidism has been lowered.) I tried different natural healing techniques to get well. I got into acupuncture, massage, chiropractic, yoga, chi kung, meditation, herbs, nutrition, and visualization. I would put acupuncture needles in myself and tape them down for the natural numbing and painkiller effects, which helped me sleep. I created vision boards for myself, pictures of what I wanted to do and how I wanted my body to look, even when sometimes I felt too ill and too weak to stand.

I wrote in my journal, went to classes, and talked with people who encouraged me to keep going. My wise stepdad Creek Hanauer told me, "Shasta, nature is so wise, nature knows how to heal itself; we just have to help it heal... Trust nature, Shasta." So this became my inner mantra, *Trust nature,* as I was trying to figure out what I needed to do to help my body heal itself.

But still I wasn't healing. I felt that life was so unfair. I had severe constipation and then acid reflux. Most everything I ate I couldn't digest. Kitchari was the only thing I could eat that did not make me feel sick. Since most foods hurt my stomach and kitchari didn't, I feel that kitchari saved my life.

By the time the doctors found my thyroid problem, I was thirty-two years old. If it hadn't been for kitchari, I don't think I would have survived. Once I was prescribed the thyroid medication, I was able to recover fully in four months.

I followed the natural remedies, ate kitchari every day, and took my hormone. It was truly a quick and remarkable recovery. In fact, after suffering from miscarriages, I got pregnant within four months of receiving the needed hormone. The endocrinologist was surprised at how well I became despite having had symptoms of hypothyroidism ever since I was a child.

Please view the before and after photo of me to the right.

My patients get very good results on the Ayurveda detox diet with kitchari. Most of them report that once on the kitchari diet, their cravings for sugar and addictive foods go away within the first week

Before   *After*

↓ Hypothyroidism (Athlethic Endurance & Weight Loss)

Lost 30 pounds
This is Shasta

and they begin to feel better and have more control over their health and well-being.

This is not surprising. Many health proponents are now stating that nutrition is more important than exercise, in fact, that nutrition is responsible for much of your health. In other words, the level of your health is not so much a reflection of how much or how you exercise, and it's not so much a reflection of your genetics. What's really important is your nutrition. I feel that most Americans have forgotten how our ancestors ate and took care of themselves as we have been uprooted from our cultures. In every culture there is a porridge or a soup known as a "recovery food."

In India, it's kitchari; in the Jewish tradition, it's chicken soup; in Mexico, it's rice and beans. In America, we have shifted away from our complex carbohydrates, the slow-burning carbs such as beans and legumes that are so important for cleansing while giving us long-lasting nutrition and "feel good" hormones. My mission is to bring back these traditional nutritional remedies that have been forgotten because we've been uprooted from our original cultures. We should also have access to the nutritional wisdom of other cultures that has sustained us for thousands and thousands of years.

My goal is to help remind you what you already know, that we are a part of nature, and that by eating more natural food we will naturally feel better. Our cravings for processed and refined foods will disappear, while cravings for healthy and nutritious foods will increase. This is our natural state and it is how nature intends us to be—vibrantly healthy.

Shasta's Pot of Kitchari Soup

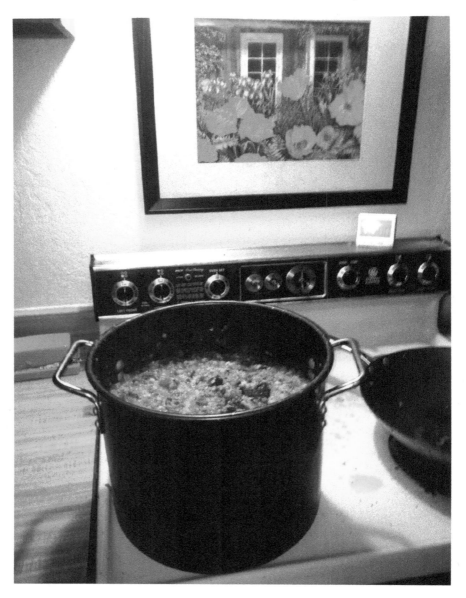

Rules for Being Human

NO MATTER WHERE you're born, to whom you're born, or how that happens, there are certain rules that a human must follow, and not by choice. Here's something written by an unknown author that I found to be truly wonderful.

1. You will receive a body. You may like it or hate it, but it will be yours for the duration of this lifetime.

2. You are enrolled in a full-time informal school called life. You will learn lessons. Each day in this school you have the opportunity to learn them. You may like the lessons or think them irrelevant and stupid.

3. There are no mistakes. Only lessons. Growth is a process of trial and error experimentation. The "failed" experiments are as much a part of the process as the experiment that ultimately "works."

4. A lesson is repeated until it is learned. A lesson will be presented to you in various forms until you have learned it. When you have learned it, you can then go on to the next one.

5. Learning lessons does not end. There is no part of life that does not contain lessons. If you are alive, there are lessons to be learned.

6. "There" is no better than "here." When "there" has become "here," you will simply obtain another "there" that will again look better than "here."

7. Others are merely mirrors of you. You cannot love or hate something about another person unless it reflects something you love or hate about yourself.

8. What you make of your life is up to you. You have all the tools and resources you need. What you do with them is up to you. The choice is yours.

9. Your answers lie inside of you. The answers to life's questions lie inside of you. All you need to do is look, listen, and trust.

10. You will forget all this…over and over again!

Life As We See It

HOW MANY TIMES have you heard the phrase "If it seems too good to be true, it probably is"? Many times we end up saying these words when something is not as good as it looks, but let me remind you that nowhere is this warning more relevant than in the domain of health and wellness. According to the Organization for Economic Cooperation and Development (OECD), Americans spend more money per capita in pursuit of good health and a fit body than people in any other developed or underdeveloped country.

Despite these efforts, we remain obese and are increasingly prone to chronic and degenerative illness. According to the CDC's most recent survey of Americans' health, released in January 2012, almost 32 percent of the two- to nineteen-year-olds and nearly 69 percent of all adults in America are overweight or obese (Hoffman & Salerno, 2012, p. 11). You will note people looking for solutions on grocery store shelves crammed with "lose weight" or unhealthy "fat-free" or the most common, "sugar-free," and vitamin-enriched products. To cure every ill we've got quick fixes—we take over-the-counter rainbow pills and pop them down to control our cholesterol and stress levels.

Despite that, we continue to feel lethargic or just plain lousy. Have you ever wondered why pills that claim to work wonders in five minutes never really work? Because they can't! Those who don't suffer from cholesterol or stress instead suffer from anxiety, allergies, colon and bowel issues, fluctuations in blood sugar, headaches, gas and indigestion, low metabolism, obesity, cramps, migraine and sinuses, skin problems, and a plethora of aches and pains. Feeling under the weather isn't considered uncommon, and we have come to accept this as our lot in life. In 2013, the combined total of those over- weight or obese reached 74 percent, according to the World Health Organization, with about half of these individuals overweight and the other half obese.

All of them are at increased risk for developing diabetes, as well as acquiring hypertension, heart disease, cancer, and strokes (Robinson, 2013, p. 18). All of these ailments, all the choices and failures we experience, could this be because of our age, gender, ethnicity, genes, or culture? Should we accept the fact that we won't always feel well and we will be prone to a host of maladies simply because of the stress brought by the physical and emotional aspects of modern life? Will we ever feel perfect? The truth is, we can—for the rest of our lives.

There are countless others whose longevity and quality of life have been completely restored thanks to the revitalizing power of healthy food and detoxification. Have you ever wondered how some people live for 100 years or more? If they recently passed on, was it just their time, or was it some kind of illness that came to haunt them? Think about it. Our planet has become increasingly polluted. And in this increasingly toxic world, we end up being exposed to dangerous chemicals every single day, with or without our knowledge.

Based on a report by the National Institute of Environmental Health Science (1999), approximately 300 billion pounds of synthetic chemicals were produced, used, and disposed of in the United States. So where are these chemicals now? In our neighbors' lawns, the dry cleaners, shampoos, face creams, household cleaners, prescription drugs, and basically everything you are using right now. Take a close look at yourself and your surroundings. Do you see anything that you would consider dangerous, like smog or smoke? Do you ingest alcohol, artificial sweeteners, caffeine, or food coloring?

Are you aware that certain foods may have been chemically stored to keep them from rotting? Don't you think that these dangerous substances can lead to degenerative illness, obesity, premature aging, or even death? Are they the reason you're constantly feeling tired or lousy? This is not to frighten you, although it may be scary to know that everything in your house and all that you eat may be the main cause for your early retirement. The reason I share this with you is to make you aware of the root cause of the numerous health problems you continue to face.

The world is a big profit market. We create the waste, pollute the environment, and then have to hire an agency to use chemicals to get rid of the waste and the pollution! Does that make sense? Probably not. But when you go to a natural-food store, you will see a variety of cleansing programs available. Some are fiber-based while others are liquid products, all dedicated to "cleansing" you from natural toxins created by your polluted environment. Moreover, some claim to free the body from toxins in just a few days—a fact that I consider an utter joke. How can anyone expect to clear away toxins that have accumulated over a lifetime by using these products for just a few days? Although some impurities may be removed, we are kidding ourselves to think that we can eliminate all of the toxins.

The food corporations are making billions on food that gives a quick lift in mood, but then leaves the body feeling depleted and even hungrier. This leads to a state of being tired but wired, where one is in survival mode even though we live in the richest continent in the world. We have been misled many times by fad diets that seem like a quick fix, rather than just coming back to the basics of eating and living a natural lifestyle with food that is whole, organic, and seasonally appropriate. As much as you enjoy a clean house, so does your spirit—your body is the house. It's very important for you to be as comfortable as possible in your skin.

It began with the low-fat diet being promoted by food corporations, the government, and the pharmaceutical industry. Even though eating low fat was an unfounded shift, it had a major impact on the health of the American people. As Americans began replacing fat with high-glycemic carbohydrates, their life expectancy began declining, despite great public health care advances. The carbohydrate issue was enforced in the 1990s when the U.S. government published its original food pyramid, which encouraged high-glycemic carbs like bread, pasta, and cereal as the largest, most important food category (Hyman, 2006, p. 49).

This book is for those who want to be comfortable, feel lively, and live the rest of their lives without any stress. And it doesn't matter if you begin the process as a pizza-eating, cigar-smoking toxin collector. It doesn't matter if you have spent half of your life tasting various wines, alcohols, processed sugar, animal fat, or anything else. This book will set things right for you. In the end, this book will leave you with a new awareness of your health, a deeper connection with your body, and the knowledge that you can look and feel wonderful all the time—for the rest of your life.

Everywhere processed foods are eaten there is an obesity problem. One-third of the world is obese, and this lifestyle and the prevent-able health diseases it creates have given new life to the publishing industry. The illnesses we face today—like fuzzy thinking, depression, anxiety, heartburn, indigestion, menopause symptoms, infertility, obesity, early aging, and increasingly common chronic conditions—have contributed to thousands of magazine articles and books and have even been highlighted on television sitcoms and reality shows. Although the aim of this exposure is to increase awareness, this in turn makes us believe that aging means illness, stress, and depression. I've heard many women in their early forties say, "Back pain and anxiety...that's because I'm aging now. Can't fight the cycles, can we!"

Yes, we can.

You are made to believe that death is inevitable—but only after a prolonged and devastating illness. Well, that's not true at all. Of course death is inevitable, but it doesn't have to be painful. This is how the commercial businesses make profit because this is the way they think. Have you ever gone through a health magazine without seeing prescription medication ads?

Do you think that just because you celebrate another birthday, you should look older, feel older, act older? Just because you have no control over the rotation of the planet does not mean that you should succumb to the forces that can be fought back. Be honest with yourself—what is the first feeling that you get when you see your friends gaining better health and vitality? Or better yet, what do you tell your friends when they complain about the symptoms of aging? Maybe "What do you expect, you're not twenty anymore"?

In one way or the other, we drag ourselves down, convinced that the cosmic alarm clock has ticked itself out. "I'm old and that's that," "I can't wear that, I'm too old," "I need rest, I'm old." Soon you'll find that these messages we create become our mantras, our litanies, and we become victims to that never-ending internal loop that limits our thinking, negates our hopes, and finally leads us to something much worse. All this can be avoided if we only take the step and believe in ourselves.

I guess by now you might be feeling silly for accepting everything that the media and commercial businesses have to offer about aging and the inevitable illness that comes with it. You shouldn't because it's not your fault; it's what you were led to believe. Every business around you—the dairy industry, processed food producers, cosmetic firms, salons, and every other business that claims to make you feel better while allowing the aging process to go on—is dependent on your belief that aging comes with lots of symptoms. After a long day of work, if you're tired and your joints ache, or if you're gaining weight, you have allergies, low stamina and metabolism, or if you're suffering from a truckload of other minor aches and pains, as far as American business is concerned, the best thing to do is to just go with it.

We must surround ourselves with people who have our best interest at heart. What's more, food processing companies make huge profits to make you believe that no matter how lousy or tired you feel, you can just grab a pizza, some French fries, and an ice cream to make your moment special at a discounted price, or with a special prize if you're a regular customer. Remember that health has everything to do with your eating habits. At the end of the month, all these corporations care about is making a profit, not about their "beloved" customers' health.

Stop believing in what the media, magazines, and television sitcoms have to offer—keep your own interest at heart. No matter what any-one says, you have the power and the ability to get up every morning free from aches and pains and full of vibrant energy. No matter how old you are, you don't have to be depressed, full of aches and pains, lethargic, or even forgetful. You don't have to become the next patient in line for consultation and medication. You have a choice. Only you can be in control of your body and nobody else. You don't have to stuff yourself with processed convenience foods that enable you to eat fast and die young. The popular American diet, no matter how cheesy and slurpy it tastes, comes with tons of health conditions that may seem inescapable, especially if you're used to it, already over-weight, or suffering from any other signs of premature aging.

But the good news is that if you give your body what it needs to repair itself from the damage, it will. And like I said before, this book is your choice to go healthy, to get rid of that unwanted "old-ness." You don't need it! Please don't get me wrong, because I expect you to make healthy choices, but the truth is you can't do everything right overnight. You can't simply read a book and affirm your decision about giving up unhealthy foods and habits. Just like you can't expect to suddenly become an expert after reading about something, you cannot make a change in a snap of fingers.

Like everything in life, making healthful choices takes time and dedication, and the best way to transform your health is to make sure that nothing written in this book goes wasted. Read this book and absorb as much information as you can and expose yourself to this knowledge, because remember, the faster you turn your health back to positive, the happier your life will be. But again, I do realize that actions speak louder than words, at least for those who lead busy and stressful lives. Whether we do it by choice or not, there are certain times in our lives that we end up making excuses to neglect our own health and diet.

So here are fourteen big excuse-busters that may relate to your life to some extent.

1. I am a mother / father and a busy person.

Let's assume that you're a working mother of two kids. If you're too busy trying to feed your family the right food, you're probably taking shortcuts on your health. If you're too busy making sure that everything else in your life is perfect, then you must reconsider your time management and your priorities. Here's something you need to know: Children and mothers who are living and eating harmoniously perform better in their social and academic lives.

2. **My community doesn't support this way of eating.**

Well, maybe it's time to change the way you look at your communities. I'm not kidding. If you live with people who do not appreciate healthy choices, you will see that their thoughts and beliefs will infringe upon your independent thought and healthy life choices.

3. **It's too expensive.**

Unless you're referring to those spas I told you about earlier or the expensive specialty items on the shelves of organic food stores, this book and the information contained· are neither expensive nor time-consuming. The ingredients in this book will not be expensive if you buy locally and seasonally.

4. **I don't have time to eat peacefully at home.**

That's something you will need to look at very carefully. Mealtimes need to be peaceful so that you can restore your health while you focus on what and how you eat.

5. **I have a stock of carbs at home. Once I finish that, I'll change. I hate wasting anything!**

I hope you realize that this type of mind-set not only costs you money, time, and energy, but it also damages your health, body, and overall environment. That's like saying, "My first aid box is full of aspirin; when I finish them, I will look at natural healing" or "I'll start breathing fresh oxygen after I run out of this secondhand smoke." The faster you realize how damaging this mind-set is, the better your options will be.

6. **I can't cook two meals, and my family will never eat this way!**

To start off with, if you want to live a healthy life while you cater to your family, you will need to take some time to prepare a healthy meal for yourself. It is advised that you make fresh servings, but if it looks impossible, you can make enough for the entire day. Even better? Gradually start weaning your family off unhealthy food choices. It may look impossible, but if you explain the benefits to your family, at least your children, they will be able to make healthy choices.

7. **Going on a vacation, I'll start when I return!**

Didn't you know that a vacation is a great time to start something like this? The point of a vacation is to balance one's life, eliminate or at least reduce stress, feel better, explore new things, rest the body, and forget everything else that made you feel old. Shouldn't this be the time to start making healthy choices too?

8. **I have a lot of health issues running in my family. I'm bound to have problems anyway.**

You must understand that a history of health problems does not mean that you are bound to get sick no matter what you do. Health problems become family problems because of the way people live and spread their habits by etching them into the generations that follow. If you want to escape this loop, you must keep your mind and body healthy by making choices that will make positive impacts on your life.

9. **I need to have certain foods or else I get irritable and hungry and suffer from low blood sugar.**

You "need" certain foods the way a coffee addict needs her big cup of strong latte. You may require them considering your need for stimulation based on your current diet, but as soon as you eat what you "need," you suddenly feel good and fully satisfied. Don't confuse this with the feeling of properly nourishing your body. Change this "need" and you'll see what feeling truly healthy is like.

10. **I'll be honest, I'm over thirty-five and I've got kids. I can never look or feel twenty anyway.**

Hogwash! Having children does not mean you must compromise your youth, longevity, leanness, or health. Motherhood/ fatherhood isn't about taking away your youthfulness; if any- thing, it enhances it. A woman's body is designed in a way that the midsection expands and contracts right back to the original size if she takes care of her health. It's not about how many times you give birth; it's about how you take care of yourself that impacts the appearance of your age.

11. **I can't do it alone. I can't focus and I'm bound to quit.**

Well, you don't have to! If you have friends, you can ask them to join you to achieve better health, and if you find your- self alone, then you have forums! There are lots of people out there who share their stories online, and you can join them. Friends don't necessarily have to be physically present, you know!

12. I'm thin and slim already. I don't need to concentrate too much. I've got no calories!

Okay, granted, being lean is somewhat associated with better health, but that doesn't mean optimum health. Thin people are prone to weariness, lousy days, and weak structures. You may look all thin and nice, but until your entire system feels like that, it's no excuse! Life is short! I want to live to the fullest!

You probably just imagined a really big meaty burger full of bacon and cheese! Well, first off, congratulations for making your life shorter. You want to live life to the fullest? How about trekking, hiking, sightseeing, camping, rock-climbing, and sky diving among other such activities? But again, how would you do that if you filled yourself with junk food and ended up being obese? Not cool! Next excuse!

13. I just can't quit. The food tastes too good!

It tastes good to your taste buds, but your digestive system is probably screaming. I do agree that a big cheesy burger tastes like heaven, but what if you found out that the heaven you taste is only a decorated image behind disasters? If this was physically possible, major junk food sellers would have packed their bags for departure! It's never too late to change your diet.

Got any more excuses?! If not, then the only way to know if the kitchari can help you heal naturally is to try it...

Introduction to Ayurveda

WELCOME TO THE enchanting world of Ayurveda! A group of holy men called *rishis* gave humankind this marvelous gift of natural health care called Ayurveda. Literally meaning "science of life," Ayurveda covers all aspects of your well-being, from simple breathing techniques to digestion. Those who know the importance and benefits of Ayurveda will agree that this is a truly holistic health system which supports you from the day you were born to the day you move on. Ayurveda greatly emphasizes the prevention of diseases and health promotion while enhancing your body, mind, spirit, and environment.

Ayurveda is an ancient form of medicine originating in India. It has many modalities such as diet, massage, herbs, meditation, therapeutic elimination, and yoga (Porter & Kaplan, 2011, p. 3414). Ayurveda is at least, if not more than, 5,000 years old, from the Indus valley where the *vedas* or oldest Ayurvedic scriptures originated. Legend has it that these vedas came naturally to a number of sages who were in deep meditation. It is believed that these sages were given the divine gift of Ayurveda based on their love and dedication to help people lead healthy and long lives. For generations, this knowledge was passed down in the form of memorized chants known as *sutras*.

There are four vedas, the oldest of which is the *Rig Veda*, which refers to the three great beings that govern the universe—*Agni* (Sun), *Soma* (Moon), and *Indra* (Wind). These in turn become what are known as the *doshas*, which govern all activities in your body: *pitta* controls digestion, metabolism, and energy production; *kapha* governs the structure of the body; and *vata* governs the movement in the body. The second veda is known as the *Sama Veda*—a purely ceremonial collection of melodies called *saman*. The third veda is called the *Yajur Veda*—also a ceremonial collection and a practical guidebook for Hindu priests who execute sacrificial acts in certain ceremonies. The fourth veda, known as the *Atharvaveda* (Stableness), contains the knowledge of Ayurveda.

In Ayurveda, the absence of disease is not considered the prime motive of a human being. In the 6th century BC, a physician named Sushruta declared that a human being is only considered healthy when his or her appetite is strong, the tissues function normally, doshas are balanced, body wastes are eliminated as needed, and when the mind and senses experience happiness. Seasons play an important role in how you react to different things because according to Ayurveda, different seasons affect your diet and your overall body and mind temperament.

Have you ever noticed that despite loving certain weather, you tend to have mixed feelings about it? For example, I love rainy season, but at times, I feel depressed because of the rain; sometimes I feel happy because I'm blessed with cool weather in a very hot country. Sometimes I just want to go out and get drenched, but often I hate the thought of wet feet. How can you explain this? We have different doshas in our body, and they change during the day and during seasons that cause emotional and psychological changes in your body. If you dive into Ayurveda, you'll notice that it understands that moving with the times and the climate is the only way to good health and a sound mind. We're all a microcosm of what's going on in our environment.

Speaking of environment, Ayurveda places great importance on environment in regards to your health. We're attached to our environment, and no matter where we go, the effects of where we stay and our surroundings don't stop haunting us. If there's brutal development in our environment, or if forests are getting wiped out or unhygienic farming practices are being carried out, we can never expect to be truly healthy. Even the food that we eat has become more hybrid than organic. Imagine the hundreds of supermarkets that sell canned food to us. If you were to can the food yourself, you would notice how fast it turns bad. Have you wondered how these supermarkets store canned goods for months? Of course they don't care for your health because these canned foods are never fresh. They are often packaged, chilled, and reheated, and the cycle goes on until it reaches your shopping bag. By that time, it contains little to no vital force. Your immune system is forced to operate on optimum capacity if the food you eat has no vital source.

In Ayurveda, immunity is known as *vyadhishamatva*, which means "disease forgiveness" and is given top priority to restore good health. Only by eating the best food will you ever improve your immune system.

You might wonder how advancement in medicine occurred if Ayurveda was the best move forward to restore health. That was my question too. There are lots of medications out there; name one disease, and you get ten different medications to cure it. The question is, if one medication is good enough to cure, is there a need for nine others? This means that none of these medications is "perfect" enough to cure that particular disease. Correct? Ayurveda has been the only system of medicine in some parts of India for thousands of years. When someone gets sick in rural India, they do not have to face hefty hospital bills to be cured. All they need are natural herbs— which are available for free in abundance!

Under British rule, the power of Ayurveda was undermined in the belief that chemical capsules and pills were faster and more effective. The poor continued to use the old and tested method of Ayurveda, while those who could afford fast treatment embraced advanced medicine and technology. Until 1947, Ayurveda was considered hogwash by people who claimed that the capsules and pills they had consumed had given them relief from their pains. Little did they know that these results were just the beginning of a lifetime of medicine consumption.

After 1947, when India gained independence, Ayurveda received full recognition as an alternate medical system. With tons of tests and assurance, nothing has been able to break the magic of Ayurveda— a medical system that is now practiced all over the world. The best part is that Ayurveda has no side effects and does not interfere with routines of busy, chemical-consuming humans.

Let's quickly look at the five elements that provide your body the energy and stamina to lead healthy lives. It is believed that the universe has given humankind three states of energy or pure consciousness to lead their lives. These energy states are known as *gunas*—which liter- ally means "ropes that bind us to the physical world." These gunas are *Sattwa guna*—a state of equilibrium and balance; *Rajas guna*—kinetic energy that allows activity; and *Tamas guna*—a state of dullness and depression, where nothing happens and rest follows. Together, these gunas form the five elements that are the primary foundation of everything material in this world.

1. Ether

In Sanskrit, ether is known as *akasha*, which comes from the root word *kas*—meaning "to radiate." This element's quality is its ability to convey energy without opposition. Ether is present in your lungs and in your colon to maintain the integrity of your body and its processes.

2. **Air**

   In Sanskrit, air is known as *vayu*, which means "movement, vibration, and gaseousness." All hollow spaces in your body, such as your throat and bones, contain air, and it serves to activate and stimulate millions of processes in your body.

3. **Fire**

   In Sanskrit, fire is known as *agni*, which means "to radiate." Fire is present is your body in the form of enzymes and your metabolic rate. From your digestive process to your thought process, fire is present all through the way.

4. **Water**

   In Sanskrit, water is known popularly as *jala*, which means "watery." Water governs all fluids in your body, as it is found in the cellular fluids in your tissues, spine, and brain. It helps lubricate your joints, moisturize your lungs and eyes, and prevent the surface of your skin from drying up.

5. **Earth**

   In Sanskrit, earth is known as *prithvi*, which is the solid state of your body. It includes your bones, teeth, and nails. Earth plays a vital role in the way you lead your life, as it provides you with firmness, strength, and stability.

Now that you know the five elements, let's look at how they affect your doshas. We learned that doshas change during the day as well as during different seasons, but let's dig in a bit more to find out what exactly they are. Doshas are the golden triangle of Ayurveda, and they are formed only when all five elements come together. There are three doshas, namely vata, pitta, and kapha, that govern a person's physical, mental, and psychological systems, and like DNA, each person has a unique combination of these three doshas.

The following chapters will provide you with a questionnaire to determine your dominant dosha. Generally, one of the three doshas will be dominant, but a few people are governed by two doshas—a very rare situation. The balance of doshas in your body is determined by a fusion of four elements—air, fire, water, and earth. Although your diet and hereditary tendencies contribute to your dosha, the amount that was allocated to you during your birth is unique to you.

Now you probably understand why two people who stay in the same house for years can never be the same! Let's take a brief look at the doshas and their characteristics to find out why certain things happen the way they do, and you'll know that after you determine your governing dosha. Remember, when you're in perfect health, all the doshas are stable, giving you peace in your mind, body, and emotions. But how you attain that state of happiness is unique to you, and sometimes nothing can compare to the happiness you get from balanced doshas in your body.

1. **Vata**

This dosha is composed of half air and half ether and is known as the primary governor. Vata is responsible for moving everything in your body—from nerve impulses, muscle contractions, and heartbeats, to moving food in your digestive system—none of which would be possible without this dosha.

When vata is in balance, you feel like a superman / woman; you gain clear thought process, free movement, and flexibility. You can imagine what happens if vata is disturbed—pains, cramps, paralysis, fear, and anxiety. The worst part is that this dosha, because of its characteristic, easily goes out of balance. If this is your primary dosha, then apart from the cramps and lousy days, you can quickly grasp and forget things as your mind is too active to stick to one point.

Your body experiences many irregularities, and sometimes you'll feel constantly hungry, other times you won't. You can easily adjust to a new environment as long as the environment changes as quickly as you adjust! You tend to be slim and tall, your eyes are quite small and active, and your hair is dry and curly. Mentally, you're active but you constantly feel the need for change as you get bored easily.

2. Pitta

This dosha is chiefly made up of the fire element with a little of the water element. Pitta governs your enzymes and hormone reactions, without which your metabolic processes would stop functioning. It regulates hunger, thirst, and body temperature and also promotes proper digestion and assimilation of both the ideas and food you eat. If this dosha is disturbed, it can lead to jaundice, conjunctivitis, fevers, and inflammation. If this is your primary dosha, then apart from burning sensations, you have a sharp intellect and matching appetite.

You have the passion, enthusiasm, and vitality to get things done the way you want them done. You're of medium build and tend not to put on weight easily. You have great focus and attention levels, and you usually enjoy studying. Although you are an ideal leader, you can be a bit obsessive if your dosha is unbalanced. Your skin is sensitive and you may have a lot more freckles and moles. You have light and silky hair, but because of excess greasiness, you have to wash it fairly often. You have a sweet tooth and enjoy cold drinks as they pacify your hot attributes.

3. **Kapha**

This dosha is made up of water and earth elements in equal measure. Kapha keeps your joints lubricated and provides your body with fluids to function and process its routine activities. It also gives luster to your skin and holds your body together. If this dosha is disturbed, you'll experience swelling, diabetes, obesity, and lousiness. If this is your primary dosha, then you're possibly an easygoing and cool person. You have strong bones and teeth; your skin is thick, preventing it from wrinkling easily.

You easily gain weight and have a hard time getting back to your normal weight. You don't like moving too much, which means that your metabolism and digestive system are slow. You take longer than others to memorize facts, but when you get there you never forget them. Your strength is the talk of town because you're capable of hard and heavy work. You're kind and loving, but because of the characteristic of this dosha, you're sometimes possessive and greedy. You like sweet and salty tastes.

That was quite a journey! You might relate to one or more of these doshas, but as I mentioned earlier, in rare cases people relate to two doshas, and every person has a unique combination of doshas. These are just starters to get you thinking about which category you fall into. In the following chapters you'll find more information about these doshas, and you will also be able to determine your primary dosha.

Ayurveda isn't an experience of a few thousand people; it's a system that has been trusted with over 5,000 years of human experience. It is truly the father of all medical modalities. This is probably the only medical system in which the healers are responsible for keeping themselves as well as their patients healthy. Ayurveda encourages using natural substances and a healthy lifestyle to vitalize the nature in you for optimum wellness in your body, mind, and spirit.

Before we move on to the next chapter, did you know that a teenager has about 10,000 taste buds? That number reduces to around 2,000 when they're eighty. You must guard what you have with the best quality of healthy food before you can no longer enjoy it or have to eat it on a doctor's advice. There's nothing in the world that can substitute for a healthy diet, because the food you eat to power your energy will ultimately affect how you feel and your ability to prevent illnesses.

In the next chapter I will ask you to take a short quiz to determine your dosha. This will be exciting, as you will see many of the visible results that determine your dosha as well as the different characteristics of these doshas. Next chapter, shall we?

Determine Your Dosha

NOW IT'S TIME to find out what your primary dosha is. Before we do that, let's take a look at a few symptoms of imbalance under the three doshas:

Vata (*Ether + Air*) **Symptoms of Imbalance**	Pitta (*Fire + Water*) **Symptoms of Imbalance**	Kapha (*Earth + Water*) **Symptoms of Imbalance**
Dry or Rough Skin	Rashes and Acnes	Oily Skin
Insomnia	Inflammatory Skin Conditions	Slow Digestion
Constipation	Stomachaches	Sinus Congestion
Fatigue	Diarrhea	Nasal Allergies
Headaches	Controlling & Manipulative Behavior	Asthma
Intolerance of Cold	Visual Problems or Eyes Sore	Obesity
Underweight or Losing Weight	Excessive Body Heat	Skin Growths

Anxiety, Worry & Restlessness	Hostility	Possessiveness & Neediness
Attention Deficit Disorder	Irritability	Apathy & Depression
Hyperactivity Disorder	Excessive Competitive Drive	Short Attention Span

Let's take the quiz together to find out your primary dosha. Tick the options that apply to you.

	Vata	Pitta	Kapha
Frame	I am thin, lanky, and slender with prominent joints and thin muscles.	I have a medium, symmetrical build with good muscle development.	I have a large, round, or stocky build. My frame is broad, stout, or thick.
Weight	Low; I may forget to eat or have a tendency to lose weight.	Moderate; it is easy for me to gain or lose weight if I put my mind to it.	Heavy; I gain weight easily and have difficulty losing it.
Eyes	My eyes are small and active.	I have a penetrating gaze.	I have large pleasant eyes.
Complexion	My skin is dry, rough, or thin.	My skin is warm, reddish in color, and prone to irritation.	My skin is thick, moist, and smooth.

Hair	My hair is dry, brittle, or frizzy.	My hair is fine with a tendency toward early thinning or graying.	I have abundant, thick, and oily hair.
Joints	My joints are thin and prominent and have a tendency to crack.	My joints are loose and flexible.	My joints are large, well-knit, and padded.
Sleep Pattern	I am a light sleeper with a tendency to awaken easily.	I am a moderately sound sleeper, usually needing less than eight hours to feel rested.	My sleep is deep and long. I tend to awaken slowly in the morning.
Body Temperature	My hands and feet are usually cold and I prefer warm environments.	I am usually warm, regardless of the season, and prefer cooler environments.	I am adaptable to most temperatures but do not like cold, wet days.
Temperament	I am lively and enthusiastic by nature. I like to change.	I am purposeful and intense. I like to convince.	I am easygoing and accepting. I like to support.
Under Stress	I become anxious and/or worried.	I become irritable and/or aggressive.	I become withdrawn and/or reclusive.

After you have ticked your options, count the numbers. The majority will be your primary dosha, while the other will be your secondary dosha. For example, out of ten if you ticked six under Pitta,mthree under Kapha, and one under Vata, then your primary dosha is Pitta and your secondary is Kapha. Good luck with finding your dosha, because the following pages contain vital information about the characteristics of your dosha and how you can prevent imbalance.

Vata Dosha Characteristics

Vata Characteristics
Helps in eliminating fetus, semen, feces, urine, and sweat
Assists with metabolism in the body and transforms the tissues
Controls important movements in the body such as respiration, heartbeat, motivation, muscle contractions, and natural urges
Relays all sensory input to the brain, motor functions
Governs nervous system

Favorable Seasons	Fall and Winter
Best Times of the Day	2am—6am and 2pm—6pm
Tastes to Avoid to Decrease Vata	Pungent, Bitter, Astringent/Light, Cold, Dry
Tastes to Increase or Balance Vata	Sweet, Sour, Salty / Heavy, Oily, Hot, Kitchari
Favorable Oils	Sesame, Almond, Apricot

Body Type

- Small frame, light and thin / hard to gain

- Coarse, dry, kinky or curly hair

- Dry, rough, darker skin

- Small eyes, whites of eyes are blue or brown

- Very large / small teeth crooked or shaded

- Performs activity quickly, can't stay idle, quick walking pace

- Low strength and endurance

- Quick minded, restless, learns fast / forgets fast, high pitch / fast voice

- Moods change quickly, tendency to worry, easily excitable, easily stressed

- Irregular hunger / digestion, tendency toward constipation

- Aversion to cold weather

- Prefers warm food / drink and eats quickly

- Spends money quickly / doesn't save

- Variable, irregular sex drive

- Light, interrupted sleep, dreams are fearful, flying, jumping, and running

Pitta Dosha Characteristics

Pitta Characteristics
Metabolism, from digestion of food to transformation of all other material
Thermogenesis—maintains the proper body temperature
Vision
Comprehension of information into knowledge / reasoning and judgment
Complexion—gives color and softness to skin

Favorable Seasons	Spring and Summer
Best Times of the Day	10pm—2am and 10am—2pm
Tastes to Avoid to Decrease Pitta	Pungent, Sour, Salty / Hot, Light, Dry
Tastes to Increase or Balance Pitta	Sweet, Bitter, Astringent / Cold, Heavy, Oily, Kitchari
Favorable Oils	Sesame, Coconut, Sunflower

	• Medium frame, medium weight
	• Thin, lustrous hair with fine curls
	• Soft, medium oily, pink to red skin
	• Penetrating eyes, whites of eyes are yellow or red
	• Small to medium yellowish teeth
	• Average walking pace, competitive
	• Good strength and endurance
Body Type	• Sharp intellect, aggressive, good general memory, medium pitch / clear voice
	• Slow-changing moods, angers easily, quick temper, likes things to be orderly
	• Sharp hunger, can't miss a meal, good digestion, normal elimination
	• Aversion to dry and hot weather
	• Prefers cold food / drink and eats at an easy pace
	• Saves money, but is a big spender
	• Moderate sex drive
	• Sound, medium length sleep, dreams are fiery, violent, and angry

Kapha Dosha Characteristics

Kapha Characteristics
Strength and energy
Moistness and lubrication
Stability to add the necessary grounding aspect to both mind and body
Mass and structure to provide fullness to bodily tissues
Fertility and virility

Favorable Seasons	Winter and Spring
Best Times of the Day	6am—10am and 6pm—10pm
Tastes to Avoid to Decrease Kapha	Sweet, Sour, Salty / Heavy, Oily, Cold
Tastes to Increase or Balance Kapha	Pungent, Bitter, Astringent / Light, Dry, Hot, Kitchari
Favorable Oils	Sesame and Olive

- Large frame, heavy, easy to gain weight

- Thick, straight / wavy, oily hair

- Oily, moist, pale, white skin

- Large eyes, whites of eyes are glossy and white

- Medium to large, white and strong teeth

- Slow and steady walking pace

- Excellent strength and endurance

Body Type

- Calm, steady disposition, long-term memory, low pitch / resonating voice

- Steady non-changing moods, slow to get irritated, very understanding, easygoing

- Can miss a meal easily, digestion can be a little slow; elimination is heavy, slow, thick, and regular

- Aversion to damp and cold weather

- Prefers dry food and eats slowly

- Saves money regularly and accumulates wealth

- Strong sex drive

- Sound, heavy, and long sleep, dreams of water, clouds, and romance

Now that you have determined your dosha, let's take a look at flavors and how they affect our bodies.

Water = Salty	
Action	Helps in softening and dissolving hardened material, lubricates intestines, great for minimizing lumps, masses, cysts, nodes, goiters
Examples	Seaweeds Cold, Saltwater Fish, Soy Sauce, Salt, Shellfish, Processed Foods
In Kitchari	Seaweed called Arame

Wood = Sour	
Action	Helps to consolidate, absorb, and bind material. Helps in stopping excessive body fluid discharge, i.e., diarrhea, enuresis, perspiration, etc.
Examples	Lemon, Pickles, Vinegar, Sour Plum, Yeast, Mayonnaise, Salad Dressings, Sour Cream
In Kitchari	Lemon Juice

Fire = Bitter	
Action	Helps in dispersing and clearing body heat, dries dampness, reduces cholesterol, and eliminates toxic heat from the blood
Examples	Kale, Chard, Coffee, Green Veggies, Mushrooms, Spirulina, Tea, Avocados, Bok Choy, Broccoli, Celery
In Kitchari	Bok Choy, Celery, Shiitake Mushrooms—neutral tonifies the qi, especially the defensive qi

Earth =Sweet	
Action	Tonifies deficiencies such as yin, yang, chi, and blood; helps reduce fatigue and anemia and relaxes the body by calming it
Examples	Yam, Honey, Corn, Grains, Meat, Molasses, Milk, Carrots, Beans, Starches, Sugar, Nuts, Squash, Fruit

In Kitchari	Pearl Barley—sweet and bland and acts like a cooling agent to the body, increases urination, relieves edema, lessens dampness, and tonifies blood and yin.
	Quinoa—although it ranks low on glycemic index it has the highest amount of protein compared to other grains,; it warms and tonifies yang and helps kidneys.
	Moong (or Mung) Beans—although this is cold in nature, it nourishes yin, stimulates hair growth, and tonifies the kidney.
	Slivered Almonds—This is neutral in action and helps increase protein in recipe.

	Metal = Spicy
Action	This increases circulation, disperses, and invigorates the body because according to Chinese Medicine, diseases come due to stagnation. Can be utilized to relieve pain, normalize irregular and painful menstrual cycles, cure edema and tumor.
Examples	Diakon Radish, Garlic, Ginger, Onions, Parsley, Curry, Mustard Greens
In Kitchari	Diakon Radish, Garlic, Ginger, Onions, Parsley, Cumin, Coriander, Turmeric, Mustard Greens

Cleanse—Nature's Way to a Healthy Life

DID YOU ENJOY taking the dosha quiz? Well, you must have noted that the only thing similar in all the three doshas are the tastes they need to increase and balance doshas—the kitchari. Before we look at what kitchari is and how you can make it without stressing at all, let's talk about cleansing your body and removing toxins and impurity. Today, nearly every culture and religious group believe that fasting rituals help remove impurities from bodies, and during that time they encourage meditation to help people focus beyond the physical realms of this world. While some follow the fasting rituals, others prefer to hold the fort and perform the cleansing process exactly as their ancient ancestors did.

Native Americans use the sweat tepees, while Japanese put their faith in communal steam baths. Cleansing rituals are not in any way spiritual or superstitious, a belief that some of us may have when we look upon these rituals. The truth is that, with pollution and our junk-food intake, we are in greater need of cleansing now than ever before. That doesn't mean these rituals emerged just because of pollution or junk food. Even when the world was a better place, these cleansing rituals were regarded as a normal, healthy, and important part of life. We must learn to listen to what our body tells us. The discomforts, pains, and fevers we experience during our lives are all signs that our body needs repair.

Apart from our environment and surroundings, we are exposed to toxins and impurities from various other sources. We can't always control our environment, but we can control the food we eat. The surprising part is that many of us believe, more than we did in the past, we are now eating more healthy foods. After all, thanks to technology, today's processed foods are fat-free or low fat, sugar-free (yet they miraculously taste sweet!), cholesterol-free, and full of vitamins, right? You need to look closer and learn how to differentiate between healthy foods and artificially healthy foods.

Before checking the price and deciding if it fits your budget, look at the ingredients—you'll notice that these artificially colored, flavored, and preserved foods are modern-day hogwash! Do fat-free or sugar-free foods attract you? While you might be very cautious about what you eat, these fat-free foods are loaded with chemicals to give you a heavenly taste and mouth appeal, filled with nothingness and void of nutrients. Your body is not benefiting from these so-called x-free foods. In fact you might as well eat the cardboard packaging!

No matter how alert you are, like I said, you are exposed to toxins and impurities from many sources. If you watch your food, your environment gets you; if you watch your environment, your food gets you. If you take care of both these sources, your lifestyle gets you. There's no escape—you need to consider a cleansing ritual. Listen to your body and you'll know that those tiny little aches and discomforts need to be repaired. So what exactly is a cleansing ritual?

Most of us are under the impression that detoxification is for those who are in rehabilitation programs to stop drug or alcohol abuse. That's not correct. To detoxify means to bring balance to our body by cleansing it and getting rid of years of accumulated toxins, inefficient fuels and impurities, and restoring it to optimal health. As much as we think about cleaning our houses, we forget that our body, too, is a house, and it, too, needs to be cleansed. Babaji says, "The body is the temple of the soul and the soul in the temple of the God."

Therefore, being healthy and having a healthy weight has these components:

1. **Chemistry**—Proper internal and external chemistry for your body type.

2. **Purpose**—realization that our body is the temple of our soul and our body is given for us to achieve our life purpose (also called dharma in Ayurveda).

3. **Nature**—trusting that we are a part of nature and that by following the way nature rejuvenates itself (cycles, seasons, flavors, etc.) we, too, can stay in a state of well-being naturally. All ancient medicines teach these principles.

Of course we treat external injuries right away, but what about years of impurities and toxins inside your body? Just because they're invisible doesn't mean they're not there. Unless you have never faced any sort of pain, discomfort, illness, fever, cramps, lousy days (and I could go on), you need cleansing. We all know the basics of first aid. If you cut your finger, you immediately clean the wound to avoid bacteria, and voila! The skin repairs itself. In a few days, you won't be able to tell that you ever had a scratch. Agreed, right?

What happens if you don't clean the wound? It becomes a habitat for bacteria and dirt and eventually becomes infected; if left untreated, the infection could become much worse and turn into a dilemma that is too large for your body's natural defenses to fight. To make it worse, it could lead to amputation or chronic diseases that you may have never imagined. Detoxification is similar to cleaning a wound to prevent it from infecting your body and causing it to give up on health altogether.

You may think you have a strong body, but the truth is that your skin, your lungs, and your digestive tract are often battered by all sorts of dangerous toxins, without you even thinking about it. It is extremely important that we understand the benefits of detoxification because if we don't clean our body from the inside, these toxins will sooner or later take charge of everything and leave us injured and full of pain and discomforts. Over time, these pains and discomforts will worsen—just like that infected finger. This isn't for the sake of filling pages; this is emphasize that you must consider detoxification.

I would feel fulfilled if you took up detoxification after reading this book. Our bodies are programmed to take care of issues they face on a regular basis. The feeling of fatigue surfaces when the body needs to build more energy so you can function well. Yawning is the body's way of telling you to stop and relax; fevers are a way of telling you there's a battle inside, "but we're on it." After working hard to make sure that you can perform your daily activities, don't you think your system needs a reward? What better way than to reward it with detoxification?

Remember, your body will only support you if you support it; if you don't, someday it will give up. Unless you're covered in plastic, there's no way you can escape pollution and environmental toxins. Whether you smoke or sit beside a smoking person, you are still injecting harmful toxins in your lungs. Your body tries to eliminate other toxins in the form of urine, feces, and sweat (if you aren't already clogging your sweat glands with deodorants and sprays). But in our advanced chemically toxic world where everyone eats processed foods, sugar, or fat-free stuff and lives on prescription drugs, our bodies collect more toxins than they can handle.

It requires help. When we talk of detoxification, we don't mean monthly schedules of detoxifying arrangement plans. We're talking about not only removing the toxins that have already made a home in your body but also keeping an eye on our future intake and avoiding welcoming new toxins in the form of processed foods.

You must stop relying on foods that provide you with no benefit. Apart from love handles and jiggly arms, you'll get nothing from junk food anyway. In this modern world, the kind of food you eat depends on many factors such as the time of day, the kind of food readily available, your state of mind, energy level, social obligations, and the intensity of your hunger. As a result, we end up eating the wrong food at the wrong time and put impurities in our bodies that do us more harm than good.

Your body is your car, and just as you don't put the wrong fuel in your car, you should not feed your body fuel that it cannot benefit from or work with. Much like plants that require sunlight and water to remain healthy, your body requires nature's fuel—nutritious foods that draw their vitamins from the earth.

These are the foods that your body needs and your cells yearn for because they are the right fuel to help you heal. Now imagine if you feasted on these kinds of food the way nature intended. You would brim with freshness, full of vitamins and minerals, allowing your body to restore its health in an optimal way. Like they say, "Easier said than done," but then again, "If there's a will there's a way," right? The food that I am about to recommend probably won't top your favorite food list, and you might not even like the taste of it when you first be- gin, but eventually, when you see its benefit, you'll begin to see how magical this stuff really is.

Unfortunately, the less you like something, the more you may need it. The process of accumulating toxins and impurities may not be difficult at all, but the process of removing them isn't always smooth and symptom-free. In fact when you first start out on your health journey, you may experience some interesting symptoms. You may feel some cleansing reactions as years of collected impurities and toxins are released into your bloodstream, urine, and feces. While some experience headaches, others suffer from slight flulike symptoms along with a bitter taste in their mouths.

Despite all these effects, you will certainly become aware of an increase in energy and a decrease in hunger. This is where I introduce God's precious food—the kitchari. There's nothing more miraculous, more benefitting, and more easy than the kitchari. The ingredients in the kitchari soup include beans, greens, onions, mushrooms, and seeds (quinoa), which are all very high-nutrient-value foods (Fuhrman, J., 2001, p. 226). High-nutrient food is measured with the ANDI scoring system, which stands for Aggregate Nutrient Density Index (Fuhrman, J., 2010, p. 28). Let's continue our journey!

Kitchari—God's Precious Food

I ASSUME YOU'RE serious about cleansing your system. Well, what better way than to take the path toward God's precious food—the kitchari, alternatively spelled as khichdi, khichri, khichdee, khichadi, khichuri, khichari, kitcheree, kitchree. Ayurvedic doctors swear by this hearty dish, made of basmati rice, *moong daal*, along with aromatic Indian herbs, and because it's super easy to make and digest, kitchari is a highly nourishing food ideal for cleansing a tormented digestive system.

According to a physician named Sushruta, a human being is only considered healthy when his or her appetite is strong, the tissues function normally, doshas are balanced, body wastes are eliminated as needed, and the mind and senses experience happiness. Kitchari provides the body with vitamins and also provides the digestive system with the break it needs to restore itself. Moreover, as part of a *Panchakarma* program—a comprehensive Ayurvedic detoxification that uses techniques such as oil massage, sweating, and enemas to evacuate toxic materials—kitchari is eaten regularly to enhance the cleansing process.

When you were asked to take a quiz to determine what dosha you belong to, you may have also noted the different tastes to avoid or increase to balance your dosha. Correct? Did you notice anything similar among these three doshas? Tastes to increase and balance your dosha, for all three doshas, include kitchari. It can become extremely difficult to follow specific diets because you might be a Vata but your partner could be a Pitta; hence you would need to prepare two kinds of dishes to cleanse your digestive systems. Apart from wasting your time over several ingredients, you would also soon give up because of the lengthy process of making this food.

Diet Therapy is a CAM therapy under the biologically based practices and entails the use of a specialized dietary regimen in order to prevent or treat a specific ailment or generally promote wellness (Porter & Kaplan, 2011, p. 3415). Kitchari is an anti-inflammatory, slow-burning, complex carbohydrate and plant-based protein medicinal soup originating from India which may include organic green mung or split yellow mung beans, quinoa, turmeric, cumin, coriander, ginger, and ghee (purified butter).

Kitchari is at the core of Ayurvedic nutritional healing. It is the main food used in Ayurvedic cleansing therapy because of its ease of assimilation and digestion (Morningstar & Desai, 1991, p. 116). Another positive finding in this study pertained to food sensitivities and allergies.

Here's where kitchari can help you. It is *tri-doshic*—meaning it is compatible with all three doshas. *One stone, two birds!* The coolest part is that it's easy and fast to make, quick to eat, and works like a charm on your digestive system. No matter what your dosha is, kitchari is the food that will enhance the cleansing process and give you the same benefits offered by the doshas' specific diets. With the fragrance of the herbs and the richness of the *ghee*, kitchari can be appreciated for its taste alone. You can add vegetables to the mix, so long as the veggies are compatible to your dosha, and have it as a nourishing soup for breakfast, lunch, or dinner.

So whether you're on vacation or busy with your day-to-day routine, kitchari is a great way to clean your digestive system from years of abuse. They say time and tide wait for nobody…there comes a time in everyone's life when they finally pop the question: "What can I do differently?" We all look at ourselves and wonder whether we've spent our lives doing the right things; maybe things could have been better. The one thing you can control is your health, and without it, you will not be able to set anything right. It all starts from YOU.

So what's all this about being healthy? Isn't health all about exercising and diet? Yep, that and much more! Exercise and diet alone are worth nothing if you're unknowingly doing and/or eating the wrong thing at the wrong time. Unfortunately Americans began eating processed carbohydrates in excessive amounts and stopped eating whole food that consists of phytonutrients, fiber, and have a lower glycemic index. Studies show that obesity will take nine years off the life of an average person (Olshansky, et al, 2005, p. 1138-1145). I do realize that in today's fast-paced world, nobody has time for themselves because they're all busy taking care of others in their family.

Admit it, you work hard (sometimes more than necessary) to raise your children, to educate them, to pay loans or mortgages, to buy household necessities; you cater to your immediate and extended family, with maybe an occasional visit to the spa. And while you do all that, your health and stamina are nowhere in the picture because all you think is "How can I make things work?" I don't blame you, but I can make your life a lot easier. If you have at least thirty minutes in twenty-four hours for yourself, then you can definitely fit in the kitchari to keep you healthy while you run your errands.

Being healthy is not an overwhelming challenge, but it is still a challenge nonetheless. And like I said, you would be able to achieve a lot more if you were healthy, because YOU come first. Dr. Fuhrman states that "scientific studies show a linear relationship between soup consumption and successful weight loss. As a weight-loss   strategy, eating soup helps by slowing your rate of intake and reducing your appetite by filling your stomach" (Fuhrman, J., 2011, p. 221).

Now, before we plunge into God's precious food, let's explore a bit and define this miraculous food.

In the West, there's no scarcity of food, from cheesy pizzas to fancy salads—a situation that gives birth to numerous disorders. Many people once thought that fasting was perhaps the best way to give their digestive systems a break from solid foods; they ended up eating more than they normally did when food was finally served!

Kitchari is a porridge from India that is traditionally prescribed during times of fasting or cleansing. According to Ayurvedic medicine, it is considered a very balanced and easy to digest, complete meal. It can be simply prepared or have endless variations, usually with a grain and legume, so it is a combination of protein and carbohydrate in a single dish. And the herbs in the kitchari have powerful anti-inflammatory properties.

Inflammation is the cause of most diseases and Kitchari has been used for 1000's of years by the Indians and by the yogi's to be healthy and have amazing longevity, flexibility, mental clarity and happiness throughout their entire lives. Now this is being discovered all over the world. Once you try it you will love it and share it with everyone you know.

The Healing Power of Ginger and Turmeric

According to Lakshmi Sridharan, PhD, practitioners of Ayurvedic medicine have been using ginger and turmeric for centuries to treat ailments such as digestive disorders, joint pain, cold, fever, cough, nausea, poor circulation, chronic respiratory illness, and neurological disorders. Unique phytochemicals in ginger and turmeric have healing properties that can treat life-threatening problems such as cancer and cardiovascular diseases, debilitating

conditions such as arthritis and osteoporosis, and many other chronic illnesses (Acharya,
A. "Use of ginger in Ayurveda, Ginger—Ayurveda's 'Root' To Good Health." Ayurveda Herbs and Spices. April 9, 2013, Kerala—Home of Ayurveda, www.homeofayurveda.org.)

Ginger's warming effects make it a natural decongestant as well as an antihistamine, making it the perfect remedy for colds. Ginger's ability to reduce PAF activity also makes the herb effective against allergies and asthma. Lakshmi's mother made soup with ginger, lentils, tomatoes, curry powder, and garlic when they had severe coughs, colds, and fevers.

Epidemiology studies show that countries whose populations consume the most turmeric also have the lowest rates of prostate cancer. India has twenty-five times fewer incidents of prostate cancer than the United States. The average intake of turmeric in the Indian population is 2-2.5g/day, providing about 60-200mg of curcumin. ("Turmeric—Nature's Chemotherapy," www.cancercompassalternateroute.com) Turmeric is also called "jiang huang" in TCM and curcuma longa. It is a member of the ginger family. It is known to be a digestive bitter and carminative and regulates and invigorates the blood.

Turmeric has many medicinal properties such as decreasing inflammation, strengthening immunity, improving digestion, and adding luster to the skin. The most unique property of turmeric is that it is spicy, bitter, and warm. Most bitter-flavored herbs are cooling, but since turmeric is warm, it helps decrease inflammation and increase circulation while protecting the digestive fire, perfect for good metabolism and digestion. According to Prasad and Aggarwal (2011), "When the turmeric rhizome is dried, it can be ground to a yellow powder with a bitter, slightly acrid, yet sweet taste."

Of course fasting is a good way to cleanse your system, but many consider it to be impractical as well as a mighty challenge to overcome. Kitchari, on the other hand, provides the same benefits as that of fasting and achieves the same cleansing goals, allowing you to continue your day-to-day activities without forcing you to faint because of hunger and/or low blood sugar! You will now realize that kitchari is not only safe, practical, and ideal, but it is also more balanced as it prevents you from starving by providing you with the right quantity of carbohydrates and protein without causing any side effects. Look at the big picture and focus on today.

Yesterday is gone, and so are all the diet failures, weight-loss spas, slimming pills, and what-not. Your future awaits you and it is only today that you can make a difference; it is today that you can start being, feeling, and living healthy.

Now to go back to our miracle food… Kitchari is a porridge from India, the Indian medicinal soup I discovered through Baba Hari Dass. Babaji eats kitchari every day. Baba Hari Dass said that the yogis in India eat kitchari as an omni food.

As I mentioned earlier, according to Babaji, the word "kitchari" is made up of two words: khe—sky and chari—walk, i.e., skywalk. Kitchari is a thick soup made of beans, rice, vegetables, and spices. This includes low glycemic index (GI) carbohydrates such as beans, vegetables; and low-GI fruits like berries, apples, and cherries (Weil, A., 2001, p. 71). The spices that are common in kitchari (turmeric, cumin, coriander, ginger) are anti-inflammatory and good for the brain, arteries, skin, organs, and more. There are fewer cases of Alzheimer's in India due to the spices.

The beans are a natural diuretic and are high in the fiber that pushes toxins out of your intestine and since they have a bitter flavor, it will decrease your sugar cravings. The yogis consider it the most pure, complete food you can eat. Baba Hari Dass said, *"The body is a boat that carries the soul on the ocean of the world. If it's not strong or it has a hole then it can't cross the ocean. So the first duty is to fix the boat."*

From a yogic perspective, food is also meant to contribute to balance and a sattvic, or clean, state of mind. So my goal with this book is to fix our boats so that we're able to cross the oceans of the world, and have fun doing it. I strongly believe that kitchari should become a staple in our American diet. Kitchari contains the whole, slow-burning carbohydrates and vegetable proteins that have been the staple of many cultures for so many years. It keeps our blood sugar stable and is high in the fiber that flushes toxins from our systems.

The antioxidants in the vegetables and the herbs and spices decrease the inflammation in our bodies that is considered the number-one cause of all modern diseases. One of my teachers, Dr. Miriam Lee, stated that "a study was done with cancer cells in a Petri dish and found that cancer cells did not grow with vegetable protein, such as beans, as they do with animal protein." The longest study on diet shows that plant-based diets tend to be healthier and give longer well-being, along with small amounts of lean, clean, organic meats and fish, perhaps due to the nutrients, vitamins, and antioxidants.

What is unique about kitchari is that it strengthens the body while detoxifying it. This is unlike most other detox cleanses which usually leave people feeling tired and dizzy. Kitchari gives long-lasting energy while alkalinizing the body, enhancing lymphatic drainage, and reducing the toxic effects of free radicals. It also can be prescribed specifically to help balance your body the way nature restores and regenerates itself. In a nutshell, kitchari:

1. Can be eaten as an omni food.

2. Is rich in nutrients that make strong blood.

3. Enhances the friendly bacteria in our gut that help fight disease, enhances our immune system, and increases the bio-availability of nutrients.

4. Helps strengthen our body's digestive system, which has been called our "second brain." Over 80 percent of serotonin is made in the intestines. Serotonin is a hormone that helps us feel full, happy, and calm—which helps us get off the roller coaster of sugar highs and lows that some people call the "sugar blues."

5. Is affordable and is gentle on the planet.

6. It can be eaten many ways such as a porridge, soup, casserole, tacos, tostadas, enchiladas, pancakes, or even blended into a smoothie.

7. It can be eaten as part of the Mediterranean diet as a lifebng healthy diet.

The Mediterranean diet is a slow burning, low glycemic, anti-inflammatory diet that has been show to help maintain normal weight, enhance memory, decrease heart disease and increase lifespan. The Mediterranean diet includes 1. Fish and lean clean organic meats and chicken, 2. Spices, 3. Vegetables, 4. Very low diary such as feta cheese, 5. Fruit, 6. Whole grains, 7. Beans, 8. Olive oil and 9. Moderate red wine.

The processed foods we have been eating have been wreaking havoc with our bodies in the form of inflammation and weight gain. Processed foods are responsible for 70 percent of American adults and 30 percent of American children being overweight (30 to 40 percent of overweight adults are known to be obese). According to the CDC's most recent survey of Americans' health, released in January 2012, almost 32 percent of the two- to nineteen-year-olds and nearly 69 percent of all adults in America are overweight or obese (Hoffman & Salerno, 2012, p. 11).

Our intestinal flora has become compromised, causing cell permeability in our intestinal walls, which lets toxins into our bloodstream. All of this causes pain throughout the body, allergies, and problems with our brains such as Alzheimer's, as well as heart disease, in-fertility, and other serious conditions. So what we're going to do is eliminate the processed foods, including foods that are known to be allergenic, for a few weeks. You will trade in the problem foods for healing, nourishing kitchari. Your body will get a break and your intestines will have time to heal.

We are going to combine Eastern nutritional practices with Western nutritional practices to allow for the best possible results. In my practice I combine Ayurvedic medical principles as well as the leading edge of Western nutritional practices. This is a program that combines the best of these traditions. In Eastern medicine, when your kidneys are weak, you will have less willpower, and you will also have more fear. When your heart is inflamed, you will be more hysterical and irrational. When your liver is toxic, you will have more anger, frustration, and depression. When your spleen is weak, you will have more confused and muddled thoughts, a heavier body, and less self-esteem. And when the lungs are toxic, you will not have as much energy, conviction, and spiritual clarity.

As you balance your organs, your emotions will become more balanced, too. During the first week of the program, you may have a hard time giving up your favorite processed foods. There may be times you want to quit because it will seem hard at first—all your processed goodies are being taken away from you. But when you get through the first three weeks, you will be amazed at your weight loss and how great you feel. You will lose your cravings for the things you're addicted to, to all the additives you've become addicted to, and you'll want kitchari instead. Kitchari will become your staple as well as your comfort food.

When we feel better, we gravitate toward the things that are good for us. When we don't feel good, it's harder to do that. This program is going to kick-start you to feel better, and you're going to prefer foods that make you feel better. Part of this is because the slow-burning carbohydrates in kitchari supply you with serotonin, the hormone that makes us feel full, happy, and peaceful. I eat kitchari as a staple every day of my life. Besides the weight loss, the benefits I have seen in my practice are just mind-boggling.

I have seen patients' triglyceride levels drop a hundred points; people whose high blood pressure went back to normal; people whose cholesterol dropped back to normal and they were able to get off cholesterol medication. I've had a woman's arm pain disappear after a couple of weeks on the cleanse program. Another woman with severe back pain reduced the pain in her back considerably by sticking to the program for three weeks. I've had patients with rotator cups so badly torn their doctor said there was nothing else but surgery, and within three weeks they were completely fine. Autoimmune rashes that several patients have had for twenty or thirty years have cleared up significantly in only eight weeks.

If I go off of kitchari and revert to my bad food habits for a few days, some of my old symptoms creep back. When I stay on it, I have the energy to do what I need to do for my practice, my family, and my sports.

I'm hoping that by doing the six-week program described in this eBook, you will choose to make healthy choices for the rest of your life. You are going to feel so good that you won't be tempted to go back to the Standard American Diet. There's nothing that can take the place of feeling slim, vibrant, and happy. And when you feel good in life, you will contribute your true, authentic gift to the world. Old habits die hard, they say, so here I am with kitchari's caloric content for those of you who like investigating ingredients and nutrient information be- fore you buy your foods!

Assuming that you use *moong dal*, brown rice, seasonings, coconut oil, mushrooms, celery, and scallions with approximately ten servings per pot, your caloric content per serving would be:

Vitamin A	19.85 mcg	Vitamin E	.63 IU	Potassium	5.66 mg
Vitamin A	240.3 IU	Calcium	73.03 mg	Riboflavin	.17 mg
Vitamin B6	.24 mg	Cholesterol	0.0 mg	Selenium	12.57 mcg

Vitamin B12	.0012 mcg	Magnesium	97.7 mg	Sodium	634 mg
Vitamin C	4.13 mg	Manganese	1.08 mg	Thiamin	.25 mg
Vitamin D	.11 mcg	Niacin	2.67 mg	Water	185 g
Vitamin D	4.6 IU	Pant. Acid	1.55 mg	Copper	.47 mg
Vitamin E	.42 mg	Phosphorous	218 mg	Iron	3.25 mg
				Zinc	1.7 mg

	Grams	Calories	Gram %
Calories		269	
Fats	4.89	42	1.6%
• Saturated	28.2	243	.9%
• Polyunsaturated	7.6	65	.2%
• Monounsaturated	8.9	77	.3%
Carbohydrates	44.9	182	68%
Dietary Fiber	9.4		
Protein	13.6	45	17%

Looks perfect, doesn't it? Now that you know the health benefits of kitchari, let's look at the kitchari ingredients and how they can assist you in your cleansing goals.

Beans and Legumes

Beans and legumes such as moong beans, split yellow peas, split green peas, green lentils, red lentils, garbanzo beans, adzuki beans, black beans, black-eyed peas, pinto, kidney, navy, and cannellini beans are a nutritious food source known for their slow release of sugar. (Meaning, beans are a slow-burning carbohydrate.) They are rich in soluble fiber (between about ten and twenty grams per cup of cooked beans, depending on the variety).

They are also high in vegetable protein and some minerals (magnesium, potassium, and folate). Beans happen to be my favorite high-fiber starchy carbohydrate. Beans are also low glycemic, which makes them a great food for most people. If you are not carbohydrate sensitive, you can enjoy any of the beans mentioned above in your kitchari. When eaten together with brown rice, amaranth, or quinoa (the gluten-free grains), you will receive the benefits of a complete protein meal.

However, some people are very sensitive to carbohydrates (for example, those with diabetes). In this case, it would be best to eat a small portion of the kitchari, perhaps a third to a half of a cup, along with vegetables and a protein. Measure your blood glucose level and see how you feel about an hour or so after eating the kitchari. Then adjust the quantity accordingly.

In summary, beans and legumes have the following health benefits:

- Slow-burning, low-glycemic carbohydrates for your energy needs,

- 10-20 grams of soluble fiber per cup of cooked beans,

- 14-17 grams of vegetable protein per cup of cooked beans,

- Rich in vitamins and minerals.

Brown Rice, Quinoa, and Amaranth

Brown rice is a slow-burning carbohydrate that is a good a source of fiber (about four grams per cup). Brown rice is also a source of manganese, thiamin, niacin, magnesium, and selenium. The ancient grains such as quinoa and amaranth are packed with nutrition. The protein in quinoa is considered to be complete, because of the presence of all eight essential amino acids (about eight grams of protein per cup).

Quinoa is rich in fiber (about five grams per cup). Furthermore, quinoa is rich in manganese, magnesium, phosphorous, and folate and is gluten-free, which makes this an alternative grain that is both nutritious and flavorful. I recommend that you use quinoa to make your traditional bowl of kitchari as it has higher protein content than any other grain.

Amaranth is also known to be rich in vegetable protein (about nine grams per cup), fiber (about five grams per cup), manganese, magnesium, phosphorous, and iron. When you combine a gluten-free grain with a bean or legume as in a kitchari recipe, you will receive the benefits of a complete protein meal that is also high in fiber. This will help move out any toxins being released from your system during your weight loss...fast.

In summary, brown rice, quinoa, and amaranth have the following health benefits:

- Slow-burning, low-glycemic carb for your energy needs,

- 4-5 grams of soluble fiber per cup of cooked grain,

- 8-9 grams of vegetable protein per cup of cooked quinoa and amaranth,

- Rich in some vitamins and minerals.

Herbs and Spices

For more than 5,000 years, herbs and spices have been an important part of Eastern cultural traditions, including traditional Chinese medicine and Ayurveda. Herbs and spices add flavor, color, vitamins, minerals, and often, medicinal properties. One of the most popular spices that has gotten a lot of attention recently is turmeric, which is widely used as an ingredient in curry dishes. Dr. David Frawely, the founder of the American Institute for Vedic Studies in Santa Fe, New Mexico, said the following about turmeric: *"If I had only one single herb to depend upon for all possible health and dietary needs, I would without much hesitation choose the Indian spice turmeric."*

The active ingredient curcumin (found in turmeric) has the following health benefits:

- Strengthens digestion and purifies the blood,

- Supports the liver and detoxification process,

- Is a powerful antioxidant, has anti-inflammatory properties, and fights cancer.

Make sure to buy the pure turmeric powder, preferably organic, as the proportion of turmeric found in a curry spice mixture may be small.

Coriander is a spice that is mildly warming. It improves blood sugar level and acts as an antioxidant. The leaf of the coriander (fresh cilantro) is known to bind with heavy metals and can reduce heavy metal concentration in the body. Cilantro is particularly helpful during weight loss, as toxins are released from fat stores. It's important to eat lots of fiber as well as cilantro to get those toxins out as soon as possible.

Ginger is known as a "universal medicine" in the Eastern tradition. Ginger helps increase circulation, supports the cardiovascular system, and promotes digestion. Ginger also helps to lower blood sugar, which means that it helps promote weight loss and rejuvenation.

Ginger combines well with onion and garlic in cooking. Cumin is known to help relieve congestion. Coriander is said to increase digestion, promote urination, and relieve gas. Ginger is used to increase digestion, relieve constipation, and reduce inflammation (Yerma & Rhoda, 2006, p. 142). Cumin, according to Eastern traditional medicine, has properties that help people lose weight.

In a recent study, the antioxidant property of cumin was found to be far more potent than Vitamin C (ascorbic acid.) Cumin has an- tidiabetic effects, helping reduce blood glucose levels. Cumin has also been found to have anti-stress properties, which will prove to be helpful when you're making changes in your diet. Herbs and spices have the wonderful property of making your diet more thermogenic. This means that they naturally help you increase your metabolism, which promotes the release of unwanted pounds.

Some spices such as cayenne pepper and red pepper flakes can also help you feel more satisfied with less food. Use the following herbs and spices fresh whenever possible: cilantro, parsley, chives, dill, fennel, oregano, thyme, sage, hot peppers, ginger, and green onions. Use the following dried herbs and ground spices liberally as well: ground ginger, turmeric, coriander, cumin, cinnamon, cayenne pepper, black pepper, caraway seeds, fennel seeds, ground cloves, Jamaican all- spice, Hungarian paprika, dried oregano, marjoram, thyme, and sage.

Vegetables

Vegetables are some of the most nutritionally dense foods per calorie. Vegetables are high in vitamins, minerals, and antioxidants. Use the following vegetables in your kitchari: onions, garlic, kale, celery, broccoli, green and red cabbage, red or rainbow chard, asparagus, beet greens, bokchoy, cauliflower, collard greens, Brussels sprouts, bell peppers, spinach, zucchini, winter squash, winter melon, carrots, sweet peas, and eggplant. When possible, try to get your vegetables in season, and from the farmer's market. Don't be afraid to talk to the farmer and try some new vegetables! (And try not to use canned vegetables.)

Healthy Fats

Healthy fats such as organic ghee, coconut oil, and olive oil have a place in your diet. One myth about saturated fats (butter, animal fats, and coconut oil) that still persists is the belief that saturated fats increase heart disease. The truth is, it's the highly processed fats—particularly the trans-fats (hydrogenated and partially hydrogenated)—that have been repeatedly linked to heart disease. Saturated fats from animal and vegetable sources provide a concentrated source of energy in your diet.

Healthy fats also provide the necessary components your body needs for proper cell membrane and hormone function. They are known to slow down absorption of food, helping you feel sated for longer periods of time. They carry important fat-soluble vitamins such as vitamins A, D, E, and K. In addition, fats are needed to help convert carotene to vitamin A, as well as help the absorption of some minerals. Coconut oil also stimulates metabolism, and increases thermogenesis.

Some vegetable oils such as corn, soy, safflower, canola, and sun-flower are unhealthy due to their highly processed nature. Many of these oils are also genetically modified (particularly soy, corn, and canola), which is another reason to avoid them. This is why I would stick to the natural, least processed fats and oils—oils that your great-grandmother may have used and fats that do not require factories, chemical extraction, and chemical processing.

In summary, the ingredients in kitchari are designed to satisfy your body's nutritional needs and your hunger, while reducing inflammation, food allergies, and levels of toxins—which will result in your body losing weight quickly and naturally.

But this is all worth nothing if I don't show you how to make your own healthy bowl of kitchari! Remember, if you add veggies, you must ensure they are compatible with your dosha.

How to Make Your Healthy Bowl of Kitchari — the Traditional Recipe

This is only appropriate if you do not suffer from metabolic syndrome and are not sensitive to sugar and carbs. Before you do anything else, you must remember to soak ½ cup of *moong deal* overnight. Remember to pre-soak the grains and beans in non-chlorinated water. Soaking the grains and beans makes them easy to digest because the water pre-digests the grains, dissolves lectins (carbohydrate-binding protein that has been linked to obesity, digestive disorders, and immune reactions), and physic acid (a compound found in the gran of grains that binds to the minerals, causing them to pass largely through the GI tract).

Another teacher of mine, who taught me most of what I know about kitchari, Darlena L'Orange L.Ac., states that "soaking the beans and grains also increases the availability of the proteins by up to 70 percent." However, you are advised to change the water a few times during the soaking process, or you may find pre-soaked and dried moong beans in your local grocery store or health food store. Assuming that you have that ready, gather the following:

Ingredients:
Ghee
½ tsp. coriander
½ tsp. cumin
¼ tsp. cardamom
¼ tsp. fennel seed, ground
¾ tsp.
turmeric 1 tsp.
salt
¼ cup quinoa, rinsed well (You can use brown or white basmati rice, but I recommend quinoa)
½ cup moong dal, soaked overnight
3 ½ cups water or vegetable broth

And don't worry, I will also tell you where to find your ingredients.

Preparation:
- Cover the bottom of the pot with ghee or oil
- Add spices and warm until fragrant
- Drain the moong daal and add them with the rice to stockpot
- Stir until coated with the spice mixture
- Add the water or vegetable broth and bring to a boil
- Lower heat and simmer for 30-45 minutes until well cooked
- Garnish with cilantro, lime, and fresh ginger!

Easy, isn't it? It hardly takes fifteen minutes to make your own healthy bowl of kitchari. So those of you who have no time for yourselves, set your priorities and set aside some time to make yourself healthy, to balance your doshas, and to look forward to a very hearty future.

Remember, you can accomplish nothing if you are not in the right state of mind, body, and spirit. The choice between making a decision and making a healthy one depends on you. I expect you to make a healthy choice, so see you on the other side!

Shasta's Low Glycemic
Kitchari Recipe For Your Body Type

This recipe is better for people with carbohydrate sensitivity. If you want to know whether you are carbohydrate sensitive, please see Appendix for your Carbohydrate Sensitive Test. Your ideal score should be 20.

Ingredients

2 cups whole *moong daal* or split yellow or green *moong daal*
1 cup quinoa (you can substitute with cauliflower rice or broccoli rice)
½ - 1 tsp. rock salt (you can even use dechlorinated sea salt)
1 tbsp. coriander seeds (finely ground)
1 tbsp. cumin seeds (finely
ground) 1 tbsp. turmeric root
powder
1 tbsp. ghee (you can use olive, coconut, or sesame oil)
3-4 cups of water (depending on how thick you want your kitchari to be) ** Use vegetables and spices that match your dosha as this will help you balance your dosha. (Determine your Dosha Quiz.) Add 1 table- spoon of ghee to your kitchari to increase the protein. I recommend adding walnuts, almonds, or even lean, clean, organic meat, bone marrow broth, or a healthy protein powder such as Garden of Life brand, especially if you score higher on the carbohydrate sensitivity questionnaire (Appendix A) or if you have insulin sensitivity or diabetes.

Preparation

- If you plan to use whole *moong daal*, make sure you soak them overnight before use. Split *moong daal* does not need to be soaked.

- Drain the water from the soaked *moong daal*.

- Take a large vessel and add 3 cups of water, *moong daal*, and rice.

- Let the ingredients boil until smooth and simmer for another 20-30 minutes, depending on the softness of the rice and daal.

- In another pan, sauté salt, coriander, and cumin seeds until they expel a fine aroma.

- Wash all the vegetables you intend to use and put them into the sauté.

- Stir the sautéed spices and add to the rice and *moong daal*.

- Mix well and serve.

This recipe, if made in ample quantities, can be refrigerated for up to three days. In East India many restaurants make the basic kitchari, just rice and *moong daal*, available to the public. Moreover, some   have gone ahead to make variations to the basic kitchari by adding other spices to contribute to its therapeutic value. If you need to eat some organic protein, you can eat wild salmon, organic chicken, grass-fed beef, and organic turkey. Here are some examples:

1. Some like to have thick kitchari, whereas others add more water to make it more like a thin soup or porridge.

2. Some add other veggies such as celery, carrots, tomatoes, on- ion, garlic, and mushrooms, and make it more like a stew.

3. Some add flavors like brass liquid aminos, salsa, or dulse (powdered seaweed).

Apart from the above information, there are a few things that you must avoid for three weeks (*Only For Modified Elimination Diet*):

Gluten (Wheat, Rye, Barley)	Dairy	**Eggs
Soy	Peanuts	Sodas
White Sugar	***Gluten-Free Oats	****Organic Corn

** **Approximately 50 percent of the American public is sensitive to eggs.**

*** **Oats need to be certified gluten-free due to cross contamination.**

**** **Organic corn recommended due to GMOs (Genetically Modified Foods).** *(For more detailed food, please see Allowed and Avoid List in Appendix D.)*

You can have:

Whole Grain Rice	Amaranth	Quinoa
Millet	Buckwheat	

What you can re-introduce at Week 4:

Add one thing at a time for four days and find out what you react to by keeping a food journal.

Nutrient Data of Shasta's Low Glycemic Kitchari

This recipe contains 243 calories total:

- Protein contains 4 calories per gram—there are 9gm in the recipe (4 x 9 = 36 calories)

- Carbohydrates contain 4 calories per gram—there are 36gm in the recipe (36 x 4 = 144 calories)

- Fat contains 9 calories per gram—there are 7gm in the recipe (7 x 9 = 63 calories)

Nutrient data opinion for weight loss 4 out of 5 stars, optimum health 4.5 out of 5 stars, weight gain 3 out of 5 stars. The estimated glycemic load 18 (typical target total of 100/day or less). The good: this food is very low in cholesterol. It is also a good source of dietary fiber, vitamin B6, folate, iron, magnesium, phosphorus, and copper and a very good source of vitamin A vitamin C, vitamin K, and manganese.

Due to the protein content being only 13 percent, I recommend adding protein to the kitchari either by drinking a protein powder (like Garden of Life protein powder as it is gluten-, dairy-, and soy-free) or something similar, adding walnuts on top of the kitchari, or eating an egg or a small amount of animal protein with each serving to balance the protein, carb, and fat ratios to be closer to 40 percent carbs, 30 percent fat, and 30 percent protein. I also recommend adding a tablespoon of coconut oil, ghee, or half of an avocado to each serving of kitchari to increase the healthy fat. I usually encourage adding chia seeds and perhaps some Braggs liquid aminos or salsa for flavoring as well.

Dr. Shasta's Mediterranean Kitchari

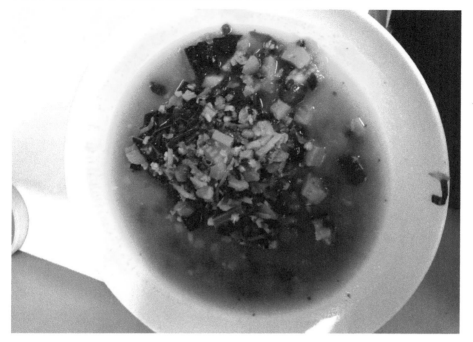

Ingredients:
4 cups of sprouted and dried moong beans
2 cups sprouted & dried quinoa (can substitute with cauliflower rice)
1 container Balti curry
1 container Turmeric powder
Dulse seaweed powder
Shitaki mushrooms
Mixed vegetables
Organic coconut oil
Braggs liquid
aminos
6 cups of water or, for more protein, 3 cups of water and 3 cups of organic chicken soup or bone marrow broth

Cook the beans and quinoa above on high flame for about 20 minutes in a large stockpot.

Preparation:
In a large skillet, add 1–2 tablespoons of whole kernel unrefined coconut oil, add a container of pre-chopped celery, carrots, and onions. Slice shiitake mushrooms, 1 entire bottle of Balti curry, 1 inch of the bottle of turmeric, 2 or more tablespoons of garlic powder, 1–2 table- spoons of kelp granules, 2 or more tablespoons of ginger, and stir while adding these ingredients to the skillet. Pour some water in to moisten the mixture and continue to simmer. After 20 minutes add 1 cup or more of quinoa to the stockpot and cook for another 20 minutes.

After the timer goes off, add the hard vegetables, like a package of julienned broccoli and other veggies, along with a packet of cut kale. Add some water if required and cook for another 20 minutes. By now the vegetables should be soft, and you can add more turmeric or whatever spices you like.

This can be left refrigerated for up to three days. Pour the remaining kitchari into 2- to 3-cup containers. Defrost when you need to eat a kitchari serving. When serving heat up with a tablespoon of unrefined coconut oil and chicken, fish, egg, or meat (if you need more protein). Garnish with salsa, avocado, chia seeds, braggs liquid aminos, almonds, or walnuts. I recommend eating this recipe within the Mediterranean diet as an ongoing optimal healthy diet.

Kitchari is very popular in India. Whenever people are sick they usually eat a very simple and easy-to-digest kitchari with split yellow moong daal, very little white rice, and very few spices, like turmeric and salt and a little bit of ghee! It is considered the chicken soup of India.

Where to Find the Ingredients:

Whole Foods and Health Food Grocery Stores
This store can provide all of the ingredients. The moong daal and

brown rice can be found in the bulk food aisle. The ghee is in the dairy section.

Trader Joe's
This store carries brown rice, quinoa, red lentils, pre-chopped veggies, coconut oil, and other organic ingredients.

Storage Suggestion
It is recommended to make at least a double batch of kitchari and store in one-cup servings in freezer containers or bags. Freeze the kitchari in the containers and remove the daily servings as needed. For example, if you plan to eat one cup of kitchari at every meal for a week, make a double batch. This will provide you with a five-day supply. Put the kitchari in a container that holds three cups. Freeze the containers and take one a day out for cooking for your meals that day. Do NOT let the kitchari sit in your refrigerator for more than three days. It will become watery and mushy.

Did you know?

- Moong daals are unique in that they supply necessary amino acids. They are rich in carbohydrates and vitamin B1 and B2, but low in fat and protein.

- Brown rice is loaded with fiber, vitamin E, vitamin B6, and magnesium.

- Turmeric contains curcumin, a compound that is both a powerful anti-inflammatory and an antioxidant. It's also non-toxic.

- Coriander and cumin are good for general digestive health. When used together they act as a diuretic.

- Cooking the spices together in ghee helps the body to better absorb them.

Okay, now that we have read all about the kitchari, how to make it, where to find ingredients, and how to store it, let me take you through my kitchari cleanse program. You no longer need to go to expensive spas and saunas; you have it all at your fingertips. The choice is, ultimately, yours.

Powerful Kitchari Cleanse Program

ALL RIGHT, WE'VE talked about a lot of things, starting from my origins to God's miracle food. We've come a long way together, and I don't know about you, but I thoroughly enjoyed your company. You may have seen thousands of diet books that claim to cleanse your digestive system, but when you open them, you'll see exotic juices and fruits that you need to buy before you even begin. Talk about the different salad colors, different fruits at different times—these books were clearly not made for the busy ones.

Times have changed so much that people are looking for ways to lessen their work. So here's my advice to you. Look at kitchari as something that you would like to try; it's not expensive, hardly takes fifteen minutes to prepare, and tastes like heaven. You're better off eating kitchari than hogging on grassy salad anyway! Remember, these salads will be present in your tummies for a temporary period of time, after which, thoughts of eating something NOW will force you to make wrong food choices.

Kitchari will fill you up adequately, it is satisfying, and you won't feel hungry. So what's this chapter about? I'm going to show you three kinds of kitchari cleanse programs—a one-week cleanse, a three-week cleanse, and a six-week cleanse—along with the kinds of foods you can add and must avoid during different seasons. For optimum health add probiotics, fish oil, chia seeds, almonds, walnuts, and flax seeds, and eat organic-food-based multi-vitamins along with triphala (use as described on the bottles) to your daily regimen. I recommend putting coconut oil, ghee, or organic butter along with chia seeds, walnuts, almonds, or flax seeds on top of your kitchari (whatever you like for taste!).

With all the three cleanses please add protein such as nuts and lean, clean, organic animal protein or healthy protein powder if you have any carbohydrate sensitivity above twenty-five. You are advised to complete the Carbohydrate Sensitivity Test that you will find in Appendix A to calculate your sensitivity level.

One-Week Seasonal Kitchari Cleanse
The one-week seasonal cleanse would include adding veggies that are in season. Eat ½ to 1 cup of kitchari three times a day with an- ti- inflammatory foods. Learn more about anti-inflammatory diets (Mediterranean diet is included) for optimum health.

Three-Week Vitality Kitchari Cleanse
During the three-week vitality kitchari cleanse, you would be required to add veggies to the kitchari that balance your doshas.

Six-Week Supreme Kitchari Cleanse
The six-week supreme kitchari cleanse aims at balancing your doshas with the modified elimination diet. Eat ½ to 1 cup three times a day for three weeks (depending on your carbohydrate sensitivity) while eliminating known allergens such as soy, gluten, dairy, eggs, non- organic corn, peanuts, sodas, white sugar, and non-organic foods. After three weeks you would need to rotate one of the above- mentioned foods one at a time every four days to see what you react to.

Remember to keep a journal to measure results. The six-week kitchari cleanse would enable you to identify any intolerances and/or allergies and help you heal any leaky gut syndrome and dysbiosis. Depending on your dosha, here's further information regarding the types of foods that you can eat and must avoid for optimum results. When coming out of cleanses, try to eat foods that are compatible with the seasons as this will help to naturally keep your dosha in balance. If you are a Vata, avoid veggies that are pungent, bitter, astringent/light, cold, or dry and focus on those that are sweet, sour, salty/heavy, oily, or hot.

Please see Appendix D for the Allowed and Not Allowed Food List. I recommend using the Ayurvedic dietary supplement preparation used in this program, called triphala. I recommend 1,000 mg of triphala every night before bed. Triphala is a combination of three herbs (fruits) that are known to be highly effective yet gentle, non-habit-forming detoxifiers. Traditional Ayurvedic physicians would use triphala as the sole herb of an entire practice due to its multiple healing properties (Yarema, Rhoda, Brannigan, 2006, p. 157).

FOOD PLAN TO BALANCE VATA DOSHA—CAN ADD			
Sweet Apples	Apricots	Avocados	Bananas
Berries	Cherries	Coconut	Fresh Figs
Grapefruit	Lemons	Grapes	Mangoes
Sweet Melons	Sour Oranges	Papaya	Pineapples
Peaches	Plums	Sour Fruits	Stewed Fruits
Sweet, Ripe Fruits	Cooked Oats Cereal	Wheat	Dairy Products
Chicken (Limited)	Sea Food (Limited)	Turkey (Limited)	Chick Peas
Moong Daals	Pink Lentils	Tofu (Limited)	Fish & Coconut Oil
Sesame & Olive Oil	Sweeteners	Almonds	Allspice
Anise	Asafetida	Basil	Bay Leaves

Black Pepper (Little)	Caraway	Cardamom	Cilantro
Cinnamon	Clove	Cumin	Fennel
Ginger	Juniper Berries	Licorice Roots	Mace
Marjoram	Mustard	Nutmeg	Oregano
Sage	Tarragon	Thyme	

FOOD PLAN TO BALANCE VATA DOSHA—MUST REDUCE OR AVOID			
**Broccoli	**Brussels Sprouts	Cabbage	**Cauliflower
**Celery	**Eggplant	**Leafy Greens	**Mushrooms
**Peas	**Peppers	**Potatoes	Sprouts
**Tomatoes	**Zucchini	Raw Veggies	**Apples
**Cranberries	**Pears	**Pomegranates	Barley
Buckwheat	Corn	Dry Oats	Millet
Rye	Red Meat	Coriander Seeds	Fenugreek
Parsley	Saffron	Turmeric	

** Can Be Eaten If Cooked With Oil

If you're a Kapha, avoid veggies that are sweet, sour, salty/heavy, oily, or cold and focus on those that are pungent, bitter, astringent/light, dry, or hot.

FOOD PLAN TO BALANCE KAPHA DOSHA—CAN ADD			
Asparagus	Beets	Broccoli	Brussels Sprouts
Cabbage	Carrots	Cauliflower	Celery
Eggplant	Garlic	Leafy Green Veggies	Lettuce
Mushrooms	Okra	Onions	Peas
Pepper	Potatoes	Radishes	Spinach
Sprouts	Apples	Apricots	Berries
Cherries	Cranberries	Figs	Mangoes
Peaches	Pears	Prunes	Pomegranates
Dry Fruits	Barley	Buckwheat	Corn

Millet	Dry Oats	Rye	Basmati Rice
Warm Skim Milk	Whole Milk	Non-Fried Eggs	Chicken (Limited)
Shrimp (Limited)	Turkey (Limited)	Almond Oil (Little)	Corn Oil (Little)
Safflower Oil (Little)	Sunflower Oil (Little)	Raw Honey	Sunflower Seeds
Pumpkin Seeds	Ginger		

FOOD PLAN TO BALANCE KAPHA DOSHA—MUST REDUCE OR AVOID			
Cucumber	Sweet Potatoes	Tomatoes	Zucchini
Avocados	Bananas	Coconut	Dates
Fresh Figs	Grapefruit	Grapes	Melons
Oranges	Papayas	Pineapples	Plums
Oats	Rice	Wheat (Limited)	Hot Cereals
Steamed Grains	Red Meat	Sea Food	Kidney Beans
Tofu	Sweeteners	Salt	

If you're a Pitta, avoid veggies that are pungent, sour, salty/hot, light, or dry and concentrate on those that are sweet, bitter, astringent/cold, heavy, or cold.

FOOD PLAN TO BALANCE PITTA DOSHA—CAN ADD			
Asparagus	Broccoli	Brussels Sprouts	Cabbage
Cauliflower	Celery	Cucumber	Green Beans
Green Sweet Peppers	Leafy Vegetables	Lettuce	Mushrooms
Okra	Parsley	Peas	Potatoes
Sprouts	Squash	Sweet Potatoes	Zucchini
Apples	Avocados	Cherries	Coconut
Figs	Dark Grapes	Mangoes	Melons
Oranges	Pears	Pineapples	Plums

Prunes	Raisins	Barley	Oats
Wheat	White Rice	Butter	Egg Whites
Clarified Butter	Ice Cream	Milk	Chicken (Limited)
Shrimp (Limited)	Turkey (Limited)	Chick Peas	Moong Daal
Tofu Products	Soybean Products	Coconut Oil	Olive Oil
*Soy Oil	Sunflower Oil	Coconut	Pumpkin Seeds
Sunflower Seeds	Cardamom	Cilantro	Cinnamon
Coriander Seeds	Dill	Fennel	Mint
Saffron	Turmeric	Cumin (Limited)	Black Pepper (Limited)

*I don't recommend much soy due to its estrogenic properties, and most of it contains GMOs.

FOOD PLAN TO BALANCE PITTA DOSHA—MUST REDUCE OR AVOID			
Beets	Carrots	Eggplants	Garlic
Hot Peppers	Onions	Radishes	Spinach
Tomatoes	Apricots	Bananas	Berries
Sour Cherries	Cranberries	Grapefruit	Papayas
Peaches	Persimmons	Green Grapes	Sour Oranges
Sour Pineapples	Sour Plum	Brown Rice	Corn
Millet	Rye	Buttermilk	Cheese
Egg Yolks	Sour Cream	Yogurt	Red Meat
Sea Food	Lentils	Almond Oil	Corn Oil
Safflower Oil	Sesame Oil	Honey	Molasses
Barbeque Sauce	Catsup	Mustard	Pickles
Salt	Sour Salad Dressings	Spicy Condiments	Vinegar

Now that you know the kinds of foods you can add as well as those you must avoid and/or reduce, below are the tables highlighting the kinds of foods you can add to your kitchari (and diet in general) as well as those that you must avoid based on your dosha to stay in harmony with the seasons.

How to Eat in Harmony with the Seasons

FOODS YOU CAN ADD DURING WINTER (FLAVOR—SALTY)			
Adzuki Beans	Clove	Lamb	Salt (Limited Usage)
Barley	Dill Seed	Lentils	Sesame Seeds
Beef Kidney	Dulse	Miso	Soybeans (Black)
Beet Greens	Egg Yolk	Moong Daal	String Beans
Blackberries	Fennel	Peas	Tangerines
Blueberries	Green Beans	Peanuts	Tempeh
Buckwheat	Hijiki	Pinto Beans	Tofu
Chestnuts	Kale	White Rice	Wakame
Chives	Kelp	Radish Leaf	Watermelon
Cinnamon Bark	Kidney Beans	Raspberries	Water Chestnuts

FOODS YOU MAY WANT TO AVOID DURING WINTER		
Alcohol	Corned Beef	Pickles
Artificial Sweeteners	Cigarettes	Pungent Foods
Bacon	Dairy Products	Recreational Drugs
Buttermilk	Frozen Dinners	Excessive Salt

Canned Vegetables	Hot Dogs	Sausage

Coffee	Oatmeal	Stimulants

FOODS YOU CAN ADD DURING SPRING (FLAVOR—SOUR)

Apple Sauce	Artichokes	Avocados	Basil
Beef	Beets	Blackberries	Black-Eyed Peas
Broccoli	Burdock	Cabbage	Celery
Chicken Liver	Chives	Coconut Milk	Cucumber
Dandelion	Gou Qi Zhi Berries	Green Lentils	Hawthorn Fruit
Kefir	Kelp	Leeks	Lychees
Moong Daal	Nori	Peppermint	Plums
Pomegranates	Quinces	Rosemary	Sesame Seeds
Sorrel	Summer Squash	Triticale	Zucchini

FOODS YOU MAY WANT TO AVOID DURING SPRING

Alcohol	Bacon	Barbequed Foods
Canned Soup	Canned Vegetables	Coffee
Fatty Foods	Frozen Dinners	Nuts & Nut Butters
Potato Chips	Pretzels	Excessive Red Meat
Salty Foods	Sausage	Sour & Sweet Foods
**Baked Foods	**Citrus Fruit & Fruit Juice	**Fermented Foods
**Spicy & Pungent Foods	**Vinegar	**Yeast Bread

** Foods to avoid during damp heat

FOODS YOU CAN ADD DURING FALL (FLAVOR—SPICY)

Adzuki Beans	Anise	Basil	Caraway Seeds	Parsley
Carrots	Capers	Cardamom	Cauliflower	Peaches
Cayenne Peppers	Celery	Chinese Cabbage	Cinnamon	Black Pepper
Cloves	Cooked Apples	Cooked Pears	Dill	Sweet Rice Congee
Garlic	Ginger	Ginseng	Grapes	Tangerines
Onions	Honey	Horseradish	Leeks	Walnuts
Licorice	Loquat	Lotus Roots	Mustard Greens	
Oatmeal	Olives	Orange Peel	Paprika	

FOODS YOU MAY WANT TO AVOID DURING FALL		
Alcohol	Beef	Cigarettes
Coffee	Dairy Products	Fried Foods
Greasy Foods	Oily Foods	Overeating
Raw Pears	Pork	Raw or Iced Foods
Raw or Iced Drinks	Sugar	**Baked Foods
**Citrus Fruit and Fruit Juice	**Cooked or Stewed Fruit	**Eggs
**Fermented Foods	**Spicy and Pungent Foods	**Nuts and Nut Butter
**Oatmeal	**Vinegar	**Yeast Bread

** Foods to avoid if experiencing thick yellow phlegm and during damp heat

FOODS YOU CAN ADD DURING SUMMER (FLAVOR—BITTER)			
All Fruits	Amaranth	Asparagus	Basil
Black Beans	Brussels Spouts	Buckwheat	Celery
Chicory	Chives	Cinnamon	Crab Apples
Cucumbers	Dandelion	Dark & Leafy Veggies	Dates
Dill	Endive	Figs	Grapes

Green Beans	Kidney Beans	Lettuce	Marrow Soup
Moong Daal	Nettles	Olive Oil	Oysters
Paprika	Parsley	Persimmons	Quinces
Raspberries	Red Beets	Red Lentils	Salmon
Squash	Spinach	Vegetables	

FOODS YOU MAY WANT TO AVOID DURING SUMMER		
Bacon	Butter	Candy
Canned Soup	Canned Vegetables	Fried Foods
Hot Dogs	High-Fat Snacks	Ice Cream
Lard	Mayonnaise	Potato Chips
Salt	Sugar	Red Meat
Saturated Fats	Whole Milk	Cigarettes

FOODS YOU CAN ADD DURING INDIAN SUMMER (OR BETWEEN CHANGES OF SEASONS) FATIGUE / ANEMIA (FLAVOR—SWEET)			
Adzuki Beans	Sweet Apples	Apricots	Bean Curd
Bitter Gourd	Congees	Cooked Vegetables	Beets
Leafy Vegetables	Carrots	Dates	Figs
Garlic	Ginseng	Grapes	Grapefruit Peel
Honey	Kumquats	Licorice	Loquat
Mandarin Oranges	Miso	Mustard Greens	Oats
Pineapple	Pumpkin	Raspberries	Squash
Stews	Sweet Potatoes	Cardamom	Cinnamon
Cloves	Coriander	Fennel	Fenugreek
Garlic Powder	Ginger Powder	Nutmeg	Orange Peel
Pepper	Sweet Basil	Cinnamon Tea	Black or Ginger Tea

FOODS YOU MAY WANT TO AVOID DURING INDIAN SUMMER OR IF EXPERIENCING FATIGUE / ANEMIA		
Candy	Celery	Dairy Foods
Raw Salads & Vegetables	Tofu	Frozen Foods
Fruit Juice	Ice Cream	Iced Water or Cold Liquids
Melon	Pork	Radish
Spicy Foods	Sugar	** Baked Foods
**Citrus Fruit and Fruit Juice	**Fermented Foods	**Spicy and Pungent Foods
**Nuts and Nut Butter	**Vinegar	**Yeast Bread

** *Foods to avoid during damp heat*

There! You now have everything you need to begin your cleansing journey. There's something else that I would like to suggest to you. After you complete your cleansing process, continue with an anti-inflammatory diet and consume highly nutritious foods which include:

HIGHLY NUTRITIOUS FOODS		
Greens	Beans	Mushrooms
Onions	Berries	Seeds

What's amazing is that kitchari includes five out of six of these highly nutritious foods! For more information, I recommend that you read the book *Eat to Live* by Dr. Joel Fuhrman. Ayurveda practitioners as well as open-minded physicians recommend detoxification to treat a host of diseases and chronic conditions including allergies, asthma, cancer, congestion, fatigue, fever, muscle pains and cramps, skin problems, and lots more. I, too, recommend the kitchari cleanse program not because I went through the pain of writing this book, but because I have seen significant results in myself as well as in my students.

See Appendix B for a Healthy Food Shopping List! Other anti-inflammatory and high-nutrient-value foods include organic

vegetables, fruits, beans/legumes, seeds, nuts, mushrooms (especially shitake), coconut and almond milk, wild Alaskan salmon, and lean, clean, organic meats. The ingredients in the kitchari soup include beans, greens, onions, mushrooms, and seeds (quinoa) which are all very high-nutrient-value foods (Fuhrman, 2001, p. 226).

High-nutrient food is measured with the ANDI scoring system, which stands for Aggregate Nutrient Density Index (Fuhrman, J., 2010, p. 28). The one thing I guarantee is that if you have been suffering from a health issue, try the kitchari cleanse program. You will note the symptoms of the illness will have diminished from your body as soon as the cleansing program is complete.

Famous activist and comedian Dick Gregory once said, *"Man does not die; he kills himself with his fork..."*

Conclusion

BEFORE YOU START your cleansing journey, I would like to say a few more things. Your body has always been showered with the wrong food, which it considers tasty and mouth-watering; therefore, before and after detoxification, you will notice that your body will crave different types of food more than it did before you detoxified. This is normal and it happens because years of built-up toxins and impurities are flushed out, allowing your body to signal you its natural preference for nourishing food. Read your body and find out what it requires apart from the kitchari to heal itself. Does it crave for a nice big red apple, or perhaps fruit cocktail? Healthy cravings will definitely lead you to a healthier lifestyle because the healthier the food, the better you will be in mind, body, and spirit.

Not only will you shed a few pounds and become increasingly active, but you will also be able to slow down the aging process. So who says all cravings are bad! Like I said before, your body has the power to heal itself no matter what your age or condition. If you give your body what it requires to maximize its power, you will experience a dramatic change in the quality of your now longer life. Within days of starting the kitchari cleanse program, lethargic feelings (what I call the 21st century syndrome) will become nothing more than a weak memory. You will no longer feel exhausted or old, because your body will constantly be upgrading its powers, allowing you to live life to the fullest. In this cleanse the aim is to improve your eating habits, lifestyle, and physical activity level.

This includes encouraging you to keep a log of your food intake, activity level, sleep, and exercise, along with meditation, yoga and qigong, and daily journaling on what you feel grateful for, successful at, and what gives you pleasure. It also includes viewing daily your "vision board" (a collage you make of what you envision yourself looking like and doing at your ideal weight). You may want to pair up with a buddy; set your health goals for each week and discuss how you did at the end of each week.

Obesity rates have tripled since 1960. This corresponds directly to two major dietary shifts in American culture. The first one was the low-fat diet being promoted by the food corporations, government, and pharmaceutical industry. Even though eating low-fat foods was an unfounded shift, it had a major impact on the health of the American people. As Americans began replacing fat with high-glycemic carbohydrates, their life expectancy began declining despite great public health care advances. The carbohydrate issue was enforced in the 1990s when the U.S. government published its original food pyramid, which encouraged high-glycemic carbs like bread, pasta, and cereal as the largest, most important food category (Hyman, 2006, p. 49).

Unfortunately American began eating processed carbohydrates in excessive amounts and stopped eating whole food consisting of phytonutrients, fiber, and with a lower glycemic index. The kitchari porridge prescribed in this program is not the traditional kitchari recipe, which usually is made up of one part moong daal and one part white basmati rice in equal proportions (Yerma & Rhoda, 2006, p. 330). The recipe used in this study has two parts whole mung (or split yellow mung) with one part quinoa (which is a seed, not a grain) to increase the protein content and decrease the carbohydrate load of the meal.

You may add many other vegetables as well as nuts, seeds (such as chia or flax), complex carbohydrates, plant protein, and slow-burning, high-fiber food. If needed, add organic meats and wild sustainable fish to increase the protein-to-carbohydrate ratio. The other important point is that the kitchari cleanse program will help decrease stress and inflammation. A recent study has found that people who feel like they have a purpose live longer.

With guided imagery (creating a vision collage of what you want to look like and do), participants stated that they visualized themselves in a healthier state, and visualized being able to accomplish things that they really enjoyed and felt were their purpose. Having a purpose in life has been cited consistently as an indicator of healthy aging for several reasons, including it's potential for reducing mortality risk (Hill, P. L., Turiano, N. A., 2014, Abstract). The National Academy of Sciences defines significant weight loss as 5 percent or more of initial body weight. This amount of weight loss is necessary to improve health conditions such high blood pressure and blood glucose and cholesterol levels.

Another method to express weight loss that is significant is a reduction of BMI by one or more points (Daly, A., Delahanty, L., Wylie-Rosett, J., 2002, p. 37). Health conditions that you once thought were there for a lifetime will begin to disappear, and your skin will acquire its natural youthful gloss, allowing you to blush every time you hear compliments. You will feel better, look better, live better, and work the way you did years ago. Your clothes will start fitting differently, and you will feel a lot like an active twenty-year-old. So what are you waiting for? The time is right; the choice is yours.

More Delightful Kitchari Recipes

Kitchari Recipes—by Cindy Fahrner

Cindy always includes 10 ounces of chopped kale to her basic kitchari recipe. She finds her kale to hold up and not become too soggy like chard or spinach.

Kitchari Soup—1 to 2 Servings
Ingredients:

1 diced onion	2 carrots, diced
4 cloves garlic, crushed	1 cup chicken broth
1″ ginger, freshly crushed	1 cup water
1 apple, diced	Veggies (carrots, kale, spinach, sweet peas)

Method:

Add to the basic kitchari / brown rice recipe onion, garlic, and ginger and sauté them together. Then use 1-2 cups of kitchari and mix with chicken broth, water, and veggies. Heat until veggies are cooked.

Kitchari Shrimp Taco
Ingredients:

Corn tortilla	3-4 cooked shrimp
Line tortilla with spinach leaves	Slice of avocado
Scoop of kitchari	Salsa

Kitchari Chile Relleno—1 chile relleno

Ingredients:

1 pasilla pepper	1 oz sliced or slivered almonds
3 oz chicken breast	1-2 oz raisins
1 cup kitchari	Shredded chicken
4 dried apricots, diced	

Method:

Peel, core, and cut the pasilla pepper in half and roast it. Cook the chicken breast—you can either barbeque, smoke, or boil it. Smoked is great, but whatever you prefer. Mix together kitchari, apricots, almonds, raisins, and chicken, and stuff each pepper half, cover with enchilada sauce, and bake at 350 for 20-25 minutes.

Kitchari Scramble

Ingredients:

2 eggs	½ cup of kitchari

Method:

Scramble two eggs, add ½ cup of kitchari, and heat through. Sprinkle salt to taste and serve hot!

Kitchari Japanese Style

Ingredients:

Cup of kitchari	2-3 ounces of shredded chicken
Steamed broccoli	
1-2 tbsp. NaGo Ginger Sesame Miso dressing (vegan, gluten-free, naturally made in SF)	

Summer Quinoa Salad (6-8 Servings)

Ingredients:

½ cup red quinoa	1 Hass avocado diced
½ cup white quinoa	½ cup minced scallion (white parts)
1½ tsp. kosher salt—divided	3 tbsp. sliced scallion green tops
1 cup seeded & diced poblano pepper	½ chopped cilantro
1 cup seeded & diced yellow pepper	4 tbsp. freshly squeezed lemon juice
1½ cup organic corn kernels	6 tbsp. divided extra virgin olive oil
1 cup organic zucchini diced	

Method:

Take a 2 qt. pot and add 1 cup of quinoa with 2 cups of water and 1 tsp. of sea salt or Himalayan salt. Bring to a boil, then reduce the heat to a simmer, cover and cook for 20 minutes. While the quinoa is cooking, shuck and shave the corn, dice the veggies, and finely chop the cilantro. Once you finish this, make the dressing by whisking 4 tbsp. of olive oil and lemon juice. When the quinoa is done, fluff it with a fork and transfer it into a large serving bowl.

Greek-Style Lemon Kitchari Soup

Ingredients:

2 cups dried yellow split peas—rinsed and soaked overnight.	¾ cups of white rice or ½ cup of brown rice
1 large chopped onion	2 tsp. cumin powder
1 tbsp. ghee	6-7 cups of water
Zest of two lemons	Juice of two lemons
Sea salt or Himalayan salt	Freshly ground black pepper

Method:

Begin cooking split peas in water and sauté onion and cumin in ghee. Add the sautéed spices to the split peas and simmer for 1 hour. Puree the soup using a blender or stick blender (easier) and add brown or white rice to the mixture. Cook white rice for 20 minutes and brown rice for 45 minutes. Finally, add lemon juice and lemon zest, salt, and freshly ground pepper to taste.

Quinoa and Black Bean Kitchari Salad

Ingredients:

2-4 tbsp. olive oil (according to preference)	1 large, finely chopped red or yellow pepper
2 cups soaked and cooked black beans	1 small, finely chopped red onion
1 regular or 2 small, chopped avocados	½ bunch of chopped fresh cilantro
Juice of two fresh limes	2 tbsp. red wine vinegar
2 cups cooked quinoa	1½ - 2 ground cumin
¼ tsp. cayenne pepper	Sea salt or Himalayan salt to taste

Method:

Mix ingredients in a bowl and serve at room temperature.

Quinoa Tabbouleh
Ingredients:

1 cup quinoa (soaked overnight)	2 cups water
1-2 cups of cherry tomatoes, halved	1 cucumber, diced
½ cup chopped cilantro or parsley	1 small, chopped red onion
¼ cup of olive oil	Sea salt or Himalayan salt to taste
Juice of 1-2 fresh lemons	About ¼ - ½ cup of olives (optional)

Method:

Cook quinoa in a covered pot and then let it stand for 5 minutes. Allow the quinoa to cool down, then add all the ingredients and mix well.

Italian Minestrone Kitchari
Ingredients:

1 cup navy beans (soaked overnight)	8 cups water
1 medium onion, chopped	2 regular stalks of celery, chopped
3 cloves garlic, minced	2 tsp. sage, diced
1 tsp. oregano	1 tsp. thyme
1 tsp. cumin	½ cup brown rice
2 carrots, chopped	2 tbsp. tomato paste
3 fresh tomatoes, chopped	2 cups zucchini, chopped
½ cup frozen peas	Small bunch of fresh parsley, chopped
Small bunch of fresh basil, chopped	Salt and pepper to taste

Method:

Cook beans in 8 cups of water, let it simmer for forty-five minutes before adding the ingredients in the following order: onion, celery, garlic, and dried herbs. Add the brown rice together with carrots, tomato paste, tomatoes, and zucchini. Remember to stir the mixture as you add the ingredients. Cook the brown rice for 45 minutes then add peas, basil, parsley, salt and pepper to taste. If desired, you can add ghee on top!

Lisa's Persian Style Kitchari with Lima Beans and Dill

Ingredients:

2 cups green moong beans	1 cup brown rice
1 tsp. sea salt	1 tbsp. coriander seeds
1 tsp. turmeric powder	1 tbsp. cumin powder
4 cups of water	2 tbsp. ghee
1-2 large onions	1 box of thawed frozen lima beans
1/3 - ½ cup dill weed, dried	4-6 large stalks of celery, chopped

Method:

Ideally, this recipe of kitchari should be flaky like basmati rice and not mushy or soupy. Soak moong beans in water for 24 hours. Drain beans and skim foam off carefully. Add the beans to 4 cups of water, cover, and cook for 15-20 minutes. Then add brown rice, salt, and cover again to cook for 45 minutes. While the rice and beans are simmering, sauté onion(s), 1 tbsp. ghee, coriander, turmeric, and cumin for about 5 minutes. Add this mixture to the kitchari and continue simmering. Then sauté celery in 1 tbsp. ghee for 5 minutes, add lima beans and dill, and add this to the kitchari.

The lima bean and dill mixture should be added in the last 5-10 minutes of cooking; celery should not be overcooked.

Christina's Kitchari Recipe *(Makes 21 cups)*
Ingredients:

1 tsp. mustard seeds	1 tbsp. ground coriander	1 tbsp. ground cumin
1 tbsp. turmeric	1 tsp. ground ginger	1 tsp. Himalayan pink salt
1/3 tsp. cayenne pepper	1 cup green split peas	14½ cups water
1 cup moong beans	6 cups water	1 cup brown rice
1/3 cup red lentils	1/3 cup green lentils	1/3 cup quinoa
2 cups celery, diced	2 cups beets, diced	4 cups red onions, chopped
4 cups red cabbage, roughly chopped	2 cups tri-colored carrots, sliced	3 cups shitake mushrooms, sliced
2 cups daikon radish, quartered and sliced	3 cups broccoli, roughly chopped	1 ear lemon, tournered and sectioned, remove seeds
4 pods garlic, minced	1 bunch purple kale	1 bunch mustard greens
3 tbsp. coconut oil		

Method:

Forty-eight hours before making your kitchari, add 1 cup of dry moong beans to 6 cups of water and soak overnight. Change water every 8 hours. Pre-measure the spices into a small bowl and set aside. Rinse rice and add to 1½ cups of water in a rice cooker. Rinse split peas and add to 4 cups of water in a medium pot over medium high heat for 20 minutes or until the beans the fully cooked. Pour beans and excess water into a food processor and puree.

Begin heating an 8-liter pot over medium high heat. Put all the chopped veggies in a large bowl and set aside. Add coconut oil to the heated pot, remove the pot from heat, and add the leafy greens, use the handles to swirl the greens until they're cooked down. Place the pot back on the burner on medium low heat.

Add the spices along with all the other chopped veggies, add 6 cups of water, stir, and cook for at least 20 minutes. While that is cooking, add the lentils and quinoa to 3 cups of water in a medium pot and cook for 20 minutes over medium high heat. Add the moong beans, lentils, rice, and quinoa to the veggie mix, stir, and cook for 10 minutes. Remove from heat and let cool. You can add more or less water for desired thickness.

Kitchari
Ingredients:

Red cabbage	Purple kale	Cayenne pepper
Mustard greens	Italian broccoli	Fresh ginger
Spinach	Celery	Cumin
Garlic with long stalk	Purple onion	Turmeric
Shitake mushrooms	Daikon radish	Sea salt—Himalayan pink salt
Lemon	Carrots	Mustard seeds
Red lentils	Green lentils	Coriander
Split green peas	Brown rice	Beets
Quinoa		

Kitchari Eggplant & Chick Pea Curry
Ingredients:

1 large eggplant, cut in half, bake at 400F for 30 minutes, cool and dice.	1 large onion

½ red bell pepper, seeded and diced	1½ tsp. cumin
1½ tsp. coriander	1 tsp. turmeric
3 cloves garlic, minced	14 oz. tomatoes, diced
2 tsp. ginger, minced	1 tsp. salt
½ tsp. cayenne	2 cups cooked chick peas
¼ cup minced cilantro	¼ tsp. garam masala
½ can coconut milk (optional)	

Kitchari Black Bean

Ingredients:

1 large onion, diced	5 cloves garlic, minced
4 stalks celery, diced	2 large carrots, diced
Black beans	Red peppers
4 tsp. cumin	2 tsp. chili powder
1 tsp. salt	Juice of 2 limes
Freshly ground pepper	½ bunch cilantro, chopped

Jeanne's Basic Kitchari Recipe for Fertility

Ingredients:

1 cup split yellow beans	1 cup red lentils
1 cup quinoa	1 tsp. salt
1 tbsp. ground coriander seeds	1 tbsp. ground cumin seeds
1 tbsp. coconut oil	3-4 cups or water or chicken/beef stock
Assorted vegetables	

Method:

Rinse lentils and peas well. In large pot add 3 cups of water or stock, peas and lentils and quinoa. Bring ingredients to a boil. Reduce heat and simmer for 20-30 minutes or until cooked. Set aside. Sauté salt and spices in coconut oil until they achieve a fine odor and flavor. Add vegetables into the sauté. Stir the sautéed spices in the peas/lentil and quinoa. Serve! Leave for up to 3 days in the refrigerator. Freeze remaining kitchari. Take out one day before needed to defrost.

Mineral Rich Chicken Bone Broth

Ingredients:

4 quarts of filtered water	*1 ½ - 2 lbs. organic chicken bones
1 heat garlic, cut in half	1 onion, cut into quarter
3 stalks celery	3 carrots, cut into 1" pieces
2 one-inch pieces ginger	1 sheet kombu, torn into strips
4 oz. fresh shitake mushrooms	½ bunch parsley
**Handful of mixed fresh herbs	2 bay leaves
Sea salt to taste	

Chicken necks, backs, and wings are inexpensive and work great

** *Includes thyme, rosemary, oregano, etc.*

Method:

Place the chicken in a large stockpot and set the heat to high. Bring the stock to a boil and skim off the froth. Add in all the ingredients, bring to a boil, then reduce the heat to low. Allow the stock to cook for a minimum of 4 hours and up to 24 hours—the longer it cooks, the better! Turn off the heat and allow the stock to cool. Strain the stock through a fine-mesh metal strainer. Place the cooled stock into glass jars for storage in the fridge (for up to a few days) or freezer for later use.

Kitchari Crockpot Chili—(Makes 33 cups)

(This can also be modified to make kitchari tacos or tostadas or burgers!)

Ingredients:

4 cups whole moong beans (soaked 24 hrs)	1 cup sprouted adzuki beans (optional)
*1.5 cups quinoa	1 tbsp. sea salt
9 cups water	2 tbsp. ghee
1.5 pkgs. mushrooms, chopped	1 onion, chopped
3 cloves garlic, finely chopped	2 tbsp. turmeric
2 tbsp. cumin	4 tbsp. chili powder
1 tbsp. paprika	1.5 jar salsa of your choice
48 ounces tomato sauce	½ cup black coffee (optional)

*If not adding adzuki beans, reduce to 1 cup

Method:

Place moong beans, adzuki, quinoa, salt, and water in a large Crockpot. Heat ghee in a sauté pan until hot. Add onions and mushrooms and sauté them until they release their liquid and start to brown. Add spices and garlic to the pan and sauté for 30 minutes or more until pungent. Add the sautéed spices to the Crockpot and stir well. Set on high and cook for 3 hours. Add the remaining spices and cook on high for an additional hour. You can add water to reach desired consistency. You can add one or more of the following:

Crushed tortilla chips	Nutritional yeast (cheesy flavor)
Black olives	Browned grass-fed ground beef

Chocolate Berry Kitchari—(Makes 16 Servings)
(This can also be made into kitchari pancakes or waffles by adding some brown rice flour, butter, and coconut milk.)

Ingredients:

4 cups split moong beans	1 cup quinoa
8 cups water	2 lbs. berries of your choice
*1 cup unsweetened almond milk	2 tbsp. turmeric
3 tbsp. cinnamon	1 tbsp. ginger
½ tsp. cloves	2 tsp. sea salt
2 tbsp. vanilla extract	½ cup pure cocoa powder (no sweetener added)
2 tbsp. coconut oil	½ cup maple syrup
1 cup unsweetened applesauce	

recipe for making your own almond milk is given below

Method:

Place moong beans and quinoa with water in a pot. Bring to a boil. Cover with lid and reduce heat to medium-low/low. Simmer for 30 minutes or until the quinoa and beans are cooked. Meanwhile puree berries in almond milk in a blender. Once the beans and quinoa are cooked, add the puree along with all the other ingredients. Simmer for 10-15 minutes. Serve with additional almond milk, if required.

You can also make kitchari pancakes by mashing up the kitchari and adding coconut or almond milk, butter, and yummy spices such as cinnamon and brown rice flour. You can even make kitchari burgers with applicable spices and brown rice flour!

Homemade Almond Milk Recipe

If you make the almond milk yourself, add the leftover nut meats to the kitchari with the remaining ingredients. You will need:

- 1 cup of almonds, soaked in water overnight

- 4 cups filtered water

Place almonds and filtered water in a blender and blend at high speed until almonds are completely broken down. Strain through a nut milk bag or several layers of cheese cloth. Squeeze nut milk bag or cheese cloth to get all the liquid out and refrigerate. Good for 3-4 days. You can also make cashew milk by following the same instructions, but replace the almonds with cashews.

Shasta's Spring / Summer Kitchari
Ingredients:

8 cups water	**7 cups chicken broth & 1 cup water
4 cups moong beans	1½ cups quinoa
¾ cup pearl barley	¾ cup millet
5 tbsp. ghee or 3 tbsp. olive oil	3 large onions
1 jar crushed garlic (4.25 oz.)	1 pound shitake mushrooms
11 tsp. cumin	11 tsp. coriander
11 tsp. turmeric	2 tsp. orange peel
3 tsp. fennel seeds	2 tsp. dried dandelion roots
3 tbsp. fresh ginger	½ bunch asparagus
1 head of cauliflower	1 cup dandelion greens
2 low sodium organic vegetable bouillon	½ bunch of large celery (8 pieces)
1 cup parsley	½ cup arame seaweed
Bragg's amino acids, soy sauce	1 lemon or lemon juice
Slivered almonds	

**If you have 7 cups of chicken broth, you can use that to substitute for 8 cups of water.

Method:

Soak beans for 14-16 hours, and then drain water. Put water in a large pot, turn to high, cook beans for 40 minutes. Add water if needed. Add quinoa, pearl barley, and millet and turn heat down to medium, cook for 45 minutes. Take a large frying pan, add ghee on high heat, cut onions and garlic very finely, and cook. Add water if needed, cook for 5 minutes. Add the washed and cut mushrooms and cook again for 10 minutes. Add water as needed.

Add more water, spices, stir, and cook for 5 minutes from medium to low. Add thinly sliced asparagus, cauliflower, celery, dandelion, and parsley to the large pot of grains and beans. Turn the heat down to medium/low. Add the seaweed and vegetable bouillon, cook for 25 minutes on low, add water as needed, and stir constantly. Let cool. Eat and flavor with Bragg's liquid aminos and chia seeds; squeeze a little lemon for taste or sprinkle slivered almonds.

Additional Info:

This soup may be eaten for 7-10 days, 3-5 times a day, with steamed or sautéed veggies and a slightly warm drink (i.e., green tea, chamomile, chrysanthemum tea). One can freeze this soup in ziplock bags and take out the night before eating. Because the carbohydrates in this soup are low on the glycemic index, individuals with carbohydrate sensitivities may eat this soup, but should add small amounts of protein with each meal (~ 2 to 4 oz.).

You can also eat room temperature apples, pears, and cooked corn tortillas. I recommend using Triphala and fish oil and a probiotic during this tonifying cleanse. I also recommend walking 20 minutes a day. You can get a ketoacid dipstick from the drugstore to make sure you are not losing too much weight too quickly. This recipe works by thermogenics increasing "digestive fire" also known as burner (warming the middle burner—metabolism). Hence it should be eaten warm.

Shasta's Fall / Winter Kitchari

Ingredients:

8 cups water	**7 cups chicken broth & 1 cup water
4 cups moong beans	2 cups quinoa
5 tbsp. ghee or 3 tbsp. olive oil	3 large onions
1 jar crushed garlic (4.25 oz)	1 pound shitake mushrooms
11 tsp. cumin	11 tsp. coriander
11 tsp. turmeric	1 tsp. orange peel
3 tsp. fennel seeds	3 tsp. dry ginger
2 large or 3 small daikon radishes	5 heads of bok choy
2 low sodium organic vegetable bouillon	1 cup fresh mustard greens
½ bunch of large celery (8 pieces)	1 cup parsley
½ cup arame seaweed	Bragg's amino acids, soy sauce
Slivered almonds	

**If you have 7 cups of chicken broth, you can use that to substitute for 8 cups of water.

Method:

Soak beans for 14-16 hours, and then drain water. Put water in a large pot, turn to high, cook beans for 40 minutes. Add water if needed. Add quinoa and pearl barley and turn heat down to medium, cook for 45 minutes. Take a large frying pan, add ghee on high heat, cut onions and garlic very finely, and cook. Add water if needed, cook for 5 minutes. Add the washed and cut mushrooms and cook again for 10 minutes. Add water as needed.

Add more water, spices, stir, and cook for 5 minutes from medium to low. Add thinly sliced daikon, bok choy, mustard greens, celery, and parsley to the large pot of grains and beans. Turn the heat down to medium/low. Add the seaweed and vegetable bouillon, cook for 25 minutes on low, add water as needed, and stir constantly. Let cool. You can eat it as it is or flavor it with gluten-free soy sauce or Bragg's liquid aminos and sprinkle it with slivered almonds for taste.

Additional Info:

This soup may be eater for 7-10 days, 3-5 times a day, with steamed or sautéed veggies and a slightly warm drink (i.e., green tea). You can freeze this soup in ziplock bags and take out the night before eating. Because the carbohydrates in this soup are low on the glycemic index, individuals with carbohydrate sensitivities may eat this soup, but should add small amounts of protein with each meal (~ 2 to 4 oz.).

You can also eat room temperature apples, pears, and cooked corn tortillas. I recommend taking the Triphala and a probiotic during this tonifying cleanse. I also recommend walking 20 minutes a day. You can also get a ketoacid dipstick from the drugstore to make sure you are not losing too much weight too quickly.

This recipe works for thermogenics (warming the middle warmer, i.e., spleen and stomach / metabolism). Hence it should be eaten warm.

Please use your own discretion when applying any of this information. It is advisable to consult with your primary care physician when taking on any new health care program.

Testimonials

"I have severe arthritis in my back and I'm in excruciating pain if I sit more than forty-five minutes, and most of the time I can't sit that long. Within those first four weeks I was sitting and working at an event for two hours and it was just amazing to me! I've also lost weight, but the pain relief has been remarkable…"—**Cindy**

"I found Way of Wellness because I was diagnosed with hypothyroidism in November, and within the past year I have gained twelve pounds without changing my diet and eating the same foods. I was wondering if something was wrong with me, so I went and got tested and was diagnosed. I wanted a natural way to heal and a natural way to feel better. Eating the kitchari has really made me feel lighter and like I have more energy. I feel that I have more clarity and I am not as exhausted as I used to be. My pH changed drastically within the first two weeks; it has now become normal. I think it was 7.8 or something like that and I think you said a normal is 7.4; it went back to normal within two weeks. So, that was good. My thyroid before I started was 6.47 and is now a 3.1, with the medication and the kitchari together with the acupuncture. I have lost a total of nine pounds and I feel enough energy to work out again. I feel like it's been a quick change too. In eight weeks to

change that much, it's pretty amazing. I am very grateful; you came at the right time."—**Monica**

"On week two I noticed that I could eat more kitchari without feeling so bloated and I wasn't craving a lot of things that I usually did. I was a soda kid. I grew up drinking soda but on the kitchari I wasn't craving it so much, some days not drinking any with no headaches. The kitchari really helped me stay full longer. I dropped two pants sizes, lost seven pounds. I feel great!"—**Jodi**

"I was diagnosed with asthma after a severe case of bronchitis. This resulted in frequent asthma attacks occurring several times a week, influenced by stress, exercise, and allergies. For most of last year I was inhaling steroids daily as well as an anti-inflammatory before exercising, and when additionally needed. The inhalers weren't treating the problem, just the symptoms. I decided to take action by going to see Shasta. She introduced me to the concept of food therapy to heal myself. I went on the kitchari diet and this resulted in major health changes for me in just a few short weeks. I have not had an asthma attack since Dec. 1, 1995, and consider my asthma to be in remission. I have also lost twenty-five pounds in the process and do not experience as much stress in my life. I feel great!"—**Andrea**

"I've had some really high-stress stuff going on and I just felt like I couldn't handle it anymore. After doing the kitchari I've lost sixteen pounds. But the biggest thing is I have clarity and I'm able to do things. I think it's getting off the sugar. I have no more cravings. I don't eat any sugar or any sweets. I'm finding as I go further into this journey, because I do feel it's a journey, that I'm in control of my life again and I think it's changed my life. I really do believe it's changed my life."—**Kerri**

"When I started the program I wanted to focus on my lack of energy, headaches, and weight loss. Upon completing the program, my headaches are less, I have more energy, my weight has maintained the same. I am more active than before. Eating kitchari has helped me balance my diet, learn my body type. I have learned to avoid certain foods that make my body more alkaline. Drinking water gives me more energy. I am getting better sleep. I used to get headaches four times a week; they are down to once a week. My belly has reduced and my tummy is much stronger. My ankles are less swollen."—**Carmen**

"I came to the class because I thought it would be the only way I could ever lose weight and that's what I really wanted to do. I've never just gone all clean, I never thought I had to do that and processed food and stuff like that, so that's the biggest thing that helped me. I'm still eating the kitchari, I'm still not eating anything processed, and this is my twelfth week. I've brought my cholesterol down so I don't have to take meds. My blood pressure has come down. I've lost eleven pounds. I'm not using canned foods. I'm eating a little bit of bread, but it has no sodium and no trans-fats, no cholesterol, and I ate kitchari for every meal and I love it. It's very filling and satisfying."—**Debbie**

"When I started the program I wanted to deal with my lack of energy and being overweight. After eating the kitchari I have more energy with no increase to my appetite, and I've lost six pounds. Upon completing this program I learned the history of kitchari and its uses. I am maintaining my healthy habits by having kitchari once a day and looking to make more healthy changes."—**Donald**

"There are no words that can describe how much you have helped me regain my self-esteem and image from being asleep for years. For

the first time in quite a few years I have been able to work in the back-
yard and not have my allergies act up!! I'd get bad bouts of asthma. I
was overloaded with alcohol, caffeine, prescription drugs, and sugar.
I weighed about 160 pounds. I'm now off the coffee, sugar, cut way
back on my prescriptions, and I've lost between seventeen and twenty
pounds, which has been stabilized for three months now!! The
kitchari cleanse really helped me detoxify my body."—**Inez**

"When I came to you, I had several problems, namely, very poor
digestion, insomnia, low energy, asthma, and anxiety. I was diagnosed
by an MD with panic disorder, which was causing most of my
insomnia. The kitchari cleanse and herbal program that you
recommended made a world of difference—I almost never have
panic attacks any- more, and I'm much calmer than I used to be. In
fact, during this same time period, my blood pressure went from high
normal to normal, another sign of my calmer nervous system. I have
also lost fifteen pounds of excess weight and have gone from a forty
waist size to a thirty-six waist size!"—**Will**

"…The surprising part is that you don't get tired of it. Energy-wise it's
amazing. I started this in January and the previous year had been a
very tough year in terms of health issues and stuff like that. It was a
struggle. Any little change would be one step forward and two steps
backward. But this is the first time since doing this program I have really stuck to it. It really feels like a lifelong change. I was also struggling
with a lot of weight gain the last fifteen year. I kind of gained forty
pounds. It's been so hard to get rid of it. I have polio so my mobility
is limited and I can't do much. I do some yoga and the swimming but
doing the kitchari I have lost some twelve pounds. I feel much lighter,
definitely more energetic…"—**Lakshmi**

"I had had chronic constipation since college; sometimes I would go for weeks at a time without a good movement. I also had candida, bloating, sore legs, and susceptibility to lots of colds and flu. I was also twenty pounds overweight. I had eaten fast foods most of my life and really was ready to make a change, especially because I wanted to get pregnant and be healthy for that. I went on the kitchari cleanse and lost fifteen pounds, and regulated my bowel movements. I feel stronger and healthier for the first time in a long time. Then, to my surprise I discovered I was PREGNANT, which really surprised me because I had been trying for four years to no avail, and wasn't sure if I would ever be able to get pregnant! Now I'm dealing with a new problem, morning sickness, but I'm very, very happy."—**Rose**

"I was forty pounds overweight after the birth of my fifth child. I was suffering from severe chronic fatigue, fibromyalgia, hypothyroid, poor memory, intense depression, and mood swings. I decided to consult with Shasta and she put me on the spring kitchari cleanse. Within six weeks I lost twenty pounds and within three months had lost thirty-three pounds. I also found much more energy and was able to do the trampoline, yoga, and participate at my child's school. It has been eight months now and I have maintained about a thirty-five-pound weight loss. I have learned that it's important to have my liver clean for everything else to work. I ate kitchari three times a day for three months (along with food) and am a firm believer in its ability to curb my sugar cravings and give me long-lasting energy."—**Mary**

"Before I started the kitchari cleanse I was supposed to be taking cholesterol meds; actually I have been avoiding them for a few years. After doing the cleanse for six weeks, I am so excited to tell you that I went to see my doctor yesterday and she told me I don't have to take my cholesterol meds and to continue doing what I am currently doing. I've also lost about twelve pounds, and my blood pressure has come down to normal. What the kitchari cleanse has done for me is *take all the guesswork out of it. I don't have to think about what to eat for breakfast, lunch, or dinner—no choices or decisions to make. I just love that!!"*—**Debbie**

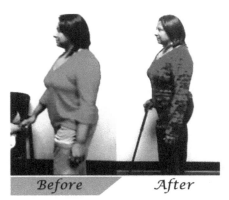

Before   After

Natural Pain Relief, Depression, Weight Loss

Lost 12 Pounds

Before   After

↓ Diabetes - dropped blood sugars 25 points to normal

Lost 6.5 pounds

Before   After

↓ Asthma, Weight Loss

Lost 25 pounds

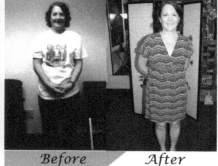

Before   After

↓ Hypertension, Diabetes & Insomnia

Lost 11 pounds

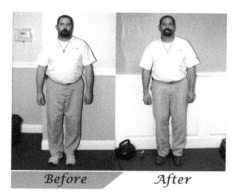

Got rid of Chronic Migraines

Lost 16 pounds

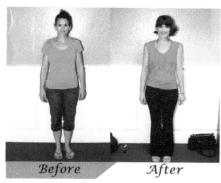

Energy, weight loss & descreased stomach ache with hashimonoto's hypothyroidism

Lost 7 pounds

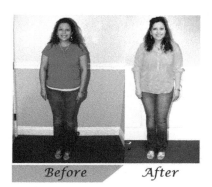

↓ Sugar Cravings & Increased Energy

Lost 6 pounds

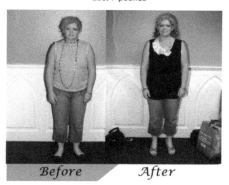

↑ Energy & Regulated homones through peri menopause

Lost 7 pounds

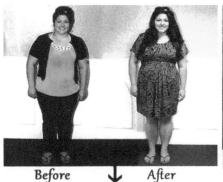

Chronic tendinitis in arms & Weight Loss

Lost 13.5 pounds

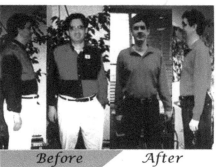

↓ Anxiety, Panic Attacks, Hypertension

Lost 15 pounds

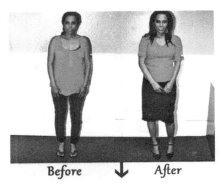

Before ↓ After

↓ Energy & Stamina

Lost 9 pounds

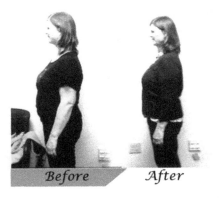

Before After

↓ Severse Arthritis, High Cholesterol

Lost 12 pounds

If they could, you can too! Good luck and God bless!

Namaste,

Dr. Shasta Ericson

Appendix A

Carbohydrate Sensitivity Questionnaire

With the increasing incidence of carb sensitivity, people must monitor their carbs—including the kitchari. Please take this test. If you score twenty points or less, you can begin the regular kitchari recipe, but if you score more than twenty points, you have to begin Shasta's customized kitchari recipe and focus on a Mediterranean diet. If your score is between twenty and forty, you should focus on more of a Zone diet, and those who score forty and above need to focus on a Paleo type of diet (beans and quinoa are okay) and eat one-half to one-third cup of kitchari three times a day with added protein. In the questionnaire below, you will find a number before the question; if it applies to you, put the same number in the blank. When you have completed the test, calculate to get your score.

Carbohydrate Sensitivity Questionnaire

(5)_____I am prone to high blood pressure.

(5)_____I gain weight around my waist easily.

(5)_____I am sometimes unable to make up my mind due to mental confusion.

(5)_____I usually feel weak, exhausted, and tired.

(10)_____I am prone to diabetes.

(4)_____During mid-afternoon, I get hungry or tired.

(5)_____I crave dessert after meals.

(3)_____If I eat carbohydrates for breakfast, I find it difficult to control my eating.

(4)_____I find it easier to lose weight by eating very little in the day than eating meals.

(3)_____Once I start eating sweets, or snacks, I find it difficult to stop.

(3)_____I would rather have an ordinary meal with   dessert than one without.

(5)_____After a full meal, I can eat the same quantity all over again.

(3)_____A meal that contains only meat and veggies usually leaves me unsatisfied and hungry for more.

(3)_____A snack of refined carbohydrates makes me feel better if I'm feeling low and/or depressed.

(3)_____If bread or dessert are served, I would rather eat them than veggies and/or salad.

(4)_____I feel tired after a meal containing potatoes, bread, or dessert, but I feel more energetic if I eat a meal containing only meat, or salad.

(3)_____Without a bedtime snack, I have a hard time going to sleep.

(3)_____If I do manage to sleep without a snack and get up in the middle of the night, I have a bite before going back to bed as it helps me sleep.

(5)_____If I miss a meal or if it is delayed, I get irritated and grumpy.

(2)_____If I'm at a restaurant, I always want to eat bread, even before the main meal is served.

Total:_____

Key Indicators

A score of 20 or less

If you scored twenty points or less, it indicates that you can perform well on a low-fat / high-complex-carbohydrates diet. You can be a vegetarian if you decide to be one or perhaps go on a Pritikin or Ornish type of diet. These are Mediterranean diets that consist of approximately 10 to 15 percent fat, 15 to 20 percent protein, and 65 to 75 percent carbohydrates by calories.

A score of more than 25

You need to follow a Zone diet that is low on sugar, sweets, alcohol, and starches but high in protein and fats. A good Zone diet consists of approximately 40 percent complex carbohydrates, 30 percent protein, and 30 percent fat.

Scores 40 and above

If you have scored forty and above, you are recommended to focus on a Paleo diet high in protein, moderate on fat, and low in carbs. In order to control blood pressure problems, you are also advised to exercise regularly as this is a vital component in any program. Remember, the higher your score, the more you are exposed to health problems and fast aging.

Appendix B

Healthy Food Shopping List

Remember not to combine any animal protein with starches such as baked potatoes, brown rice, or other grains.

Quinoa (steamed or sprouted)	Millet (steamed or sprouted)
Amaranth (steamed or sprouted)	Quinoa pastas
Steamed legumes (lentils, beans, garbanzo)	Peas
Brown rice products (rice cakes, pastas)	Buckwheat (steamed of sprouted)
Gluten-free pastas	Brown rice
Non GMO corn products	Beans
Cooked whole potatoes	Sweet potatoes
Yams, squashes, pumpkins	Whole grain bread (gluten-free preferred)
Organic eggs	Egg whites
Chicken	Fish
Turkey	Goat's cheese (raw preferred)
Goat's milk (raw preferred)	Goat's sour cream (raw preferred)
Goat's cottage cheese (raw preferred)	Steamed veggies
Fruits	Nuts

Seeds	Dry fruits
Vegetables	Avocadoes
Olives	Flax crackers
Natural nut or seed oil	Olive oil
Coconut oil	Apple cider vinegar
Seaweeds	Sprouts
Legumes	Fermented foods
Preserved veggies in oil	Bee products (honey, pollen, royal jelly)
Dehydrated foods	Super foods (goji berries, maca, acai, etc.)
Algaes	Raw cacao
Salt (sea salt, Himalayan salt)	Whole spices and herbs

Appendix C

Results and Conclusions of a
Six-Week Kitchari Cleanse Program Led by Shasta

Objective Findings: One hundred percent of the eleven participants lost weight, between 0.5 pounds and 17.5 pounds. Average weight loss for the participants was 7.68 pounds; however, the participants who did the three-week modified elimination diet 100 percent had a weight loss of an average of 9.93 pounds. The average of their blood pressure readings stayed about the same (119/76 before to 118/76 after); however, one participant who suffered from hypothyroidism and fatigue had an increase from 95/67 to 121/77 and reported a great increase in energy. The waist circumference dropped in five out of seven of the participants, two stayed the same, and four out of the eleven did not provide complete data so were not counted.

Body composition analysis using a body fat caliper showed a drop of 16.86 points (from 98 to 81.14). The participant's body mass index dropped an average of 1.32 (from 30.10 to 28.78). The saliva pH stayed about the same (average of 6.77 to 6.89); however, one participant who complained of severe migraines had a starting pH of 5 and after the program went up into normal range of 7.2, and the migraines were nonexistent. Their waist-hip ratio (WHR) measurements showed a drop in six out of seven (one of the seven stayed the same), and four participants were immeasurable due to missing data.

Of the six that went down, two went from an unacceptable level (greater than 0.8) to an acceptable level (less than 0.8). Nine out of the eleven participants reported having food intolerance, primarily to gluten. No significant study-related adverse events were reported. The participants who did the customized kitchari cleanse for their body type along with the three-week modified elimination diet 100 percent (did not eat any of the excluded known food allergens) and even the participants who partially did this were able to identify underlying sensitivities that were contributing to inflammation in their body, and thus weight gain.

All participants but two reported food sensitivities ranging from gluten as the highest, then dairy, then eggs, and lastly sugar. This is an important factor for weight-loss programs, as weight-management plans should be customized for the individual. It is estimated that at least 1 percent of the U.S. population has celiac disease, 15 percent or more are gluten-intolerant, and many people are lactose intolerant—this speaks to the need for personalization (D'Adamo, et al, 2011, p. 78).

There were three participants who stated that the one cup of kitchari three times a day was too much for them. One of these participants had severe diabetes. She stated that her blood sugars went up; however, upon interviewing her, she mentioned that she had added dried fruit as a snack. Dried fruit is very high in sugar (high GI-index); therefore, her assertion is unclear. The other participant, who also had diabetes, reduced from one cup of kitchari down to half a cup.

She actually ended up losing 6.5 pounds and brought her blood sugars down to normal for the first time in years. The third participant reported constipation and went to her physician, who found a fibroid the size of a thirteen-week fetus in her uterus. He proceeded to do a full hysterectomy as the participant had been suffering from very heavy periods. The participant kept up with the kitchari porridge and reported feeling much better overall and lost 12½ pounds by the end of the six weeks.

Appendix D

FOOD GROUP	ALLOWED	AVOID
Meat, Fish, Poultry	Chicken, turkey, lamb. All legumes, dried peas and lentils. Coldwater fish such as salmon, halibut and mackerel.	Processed meats, cold cuts, frankfurter, sausage, canned sausage, canned meats and eggs.
Dairy Products	Milk substitutes such as rice milk, nut milks, and ghee.	Milk, cheese, ice cream, cream, non-dairy creamers.
Starch	White or sweet potato, brown rice, tapioca, buckwheat and gluten-free products.	All gluten-containing products, including gluten-containing pasta.
Soups	Clear, vegetable-based broth, homemade vegetarian soups.	Canned or cream soups.
Vegetables	All vegetables, preferably fresh, frozen or freshly juiced.	Creamed or in casseroles.
Beverages	Vegetable juices, water, herbal teas, occasional glass of red wine.	Milk, coffee, tea, cocoa, Postum, alcoholic beverages, soda pop, sweetened beverages, citrus.

Bread/Cereals	Rice, buckwheat, millet, potato flour, tapioca, arrowroot or gluten-free flour-based products.	All made from wheat, oat, spelt, kamut, rye, barley, amaranth, quinoa, or gluten-containing products.
Fruits	Unsweetened fresh or frozen.	Fruit drinks, aides, or dried fruit.
Fats/Oils/Nuts	Cold/expeller pressed, unrefined, coconut, flax, or olive oils, ghee, sesame, flax pumpkin, squash seeds/butters, salad dressings made from allowed ingredients, almonds, cashews, pecans, and walnuts.	Margarine, shortening, un-clarified butter, refined oils, peanuts, salad dressings and spreads.

References

Daly, A., Delahanty, L., Wylie-Rosett, J. (2002). *101 weight loss tips for people with diabetes.* Alexandria, VI: America Diabetes Association.

Fuhrman, J. (2010). *Eat right America: Enjoy a whole life.* United States: Nutritional Excellence, LLC.

Fuhrman, J. (2011). *Eat to Live: The amazing nutrient-rich program for fast and sustained weight loss.* New York, NY: Little, Brown Press.

Hill, P., Turiano, N. A. (2014). Purpose in life as a predictor of mortality across adulthood. *Psychological Science,* May 8, 2014.

Hoffman, J., Salerno, J. A. (2012). *The weight of the nation: To win we have to lose.* New York, NY: St. Martin's Press.

Hyman, M., (2006). *Ultra Metabolism: The simple plan for automatic weight loss,* NY: Atria Books.

Morningstar, A., Desai, U. (1991). *The ayurvedic cookbook: A personalized guide to good nutrition and health.* Wilmot, WI: Lotus Press.

Olshansky, S., Passaro, D., Hershow, R., Layden, J., Carnes, B., Brody, J. Hayflick, L., Butler, R., Allison, D., Ludwig, D. (2005). A potential decline in life expectancy in the United States in the 21st century. *New England Journal of Medicine, 352* (11), 1138-1145.

Porter, R. S., Kaplan, J. L. (Eds.). (2011). *The Merck manual: Of diagnosis and therapy: Nineteenth edition.* Whitehouse Station, NJ: Merck Sharp & Dohme Corp.

Prasad, S. & Aggarwal, B. B. (2011). Herbal medicine: Bimolecular and clinical aspects. 2nd edition. Boca Raton, FL: CRC Press.

Robinson, B. H. (2013). The greatest health crisis in America. *Acupuncture Today, 14* (3), 1-24.

Ulbricht, C., D'Adamo, C., & Ernst, E. (2011). Roundtable discussion: An integrative approach to healthy body weight. *Alternative and Complementary Therapies, 17* (2), 76-83.

Weil, A. (2001). *Eating well for optimum health: The essential guide to bringing health and pleasure back to eating.* New York, NY: HarperCollins Publishers Inc.

Yarema, T., Rhoda, D., Brannigan, J. (2006). *Eat taste heal: An ayurvedic guidebook and cookbook for modern living.* Kapaa, HI: Five-Element Press.

CPSIA information can be obtained
at www.ICGtesting.com
Printed in the USA
JSHW010719240520
5812JS00005B/44

9 781647 490638